The Ultimate Simple Keto Cookbook

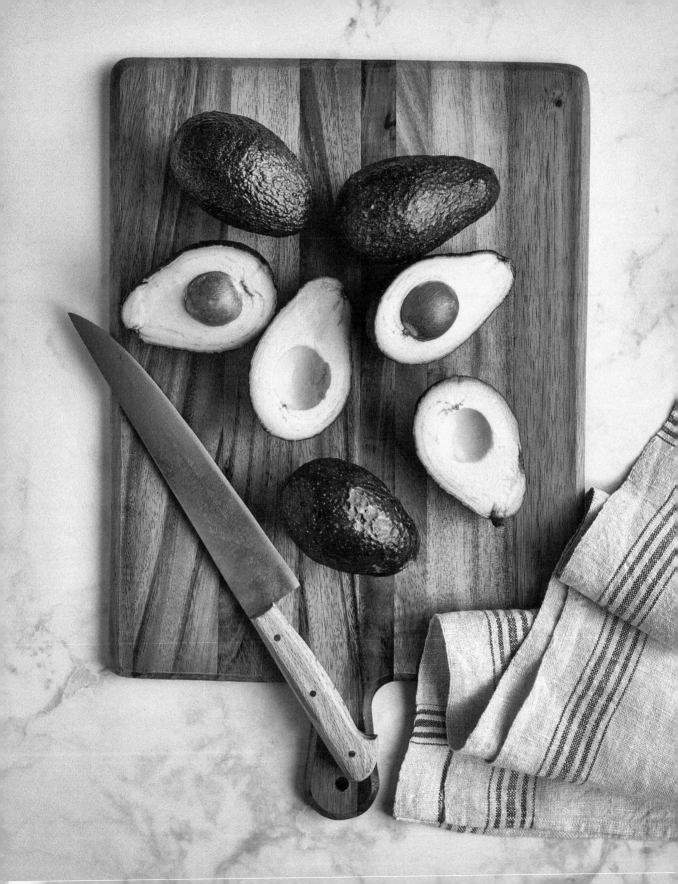

THE ULTIMATE
Simple Keto Cookbook

EASY KETOGENIC DIET RECIPES

Emilie Bailey

ROCKRIDGE
PRESS

For general information on our other products and services or to obtain technical support, please contact our Customer Care Department within the United States at (866) 744-2665, or outside the United States at (510) 253-0500.

Rockridge Press publishes its books in a variety of electronic and print formats. Some content that appears in print may not be available in electronic books, and vice versa.

Interior and Cover Designer: Diana Haas
Art Producer: Tom Hood
Editor: Justin Hartung
Production Editor: Rachel Taenzler
Production Manager: Michael Kay

Photography © Hélène Dujardin, 2021, with food styling by Anna Hampton, cover & pp ii, vi, ix, x, 12, 33, 35, 49, 56, 60, 78, 90, 100, 115, 128, 149, 156, 160, 174, 189, 194; Laura Flippen with food styling by Cole Church, pp 27, 40, 69, 176; Nadine Greeff, pp 87, 118, 139; Annie Martin with food styling by Oscar Molinar, p. 172

ISBN: Print 978-1-64876-411-0 | eBook 978-1-64876-412-7

R0

For my Granny—I will always remember.

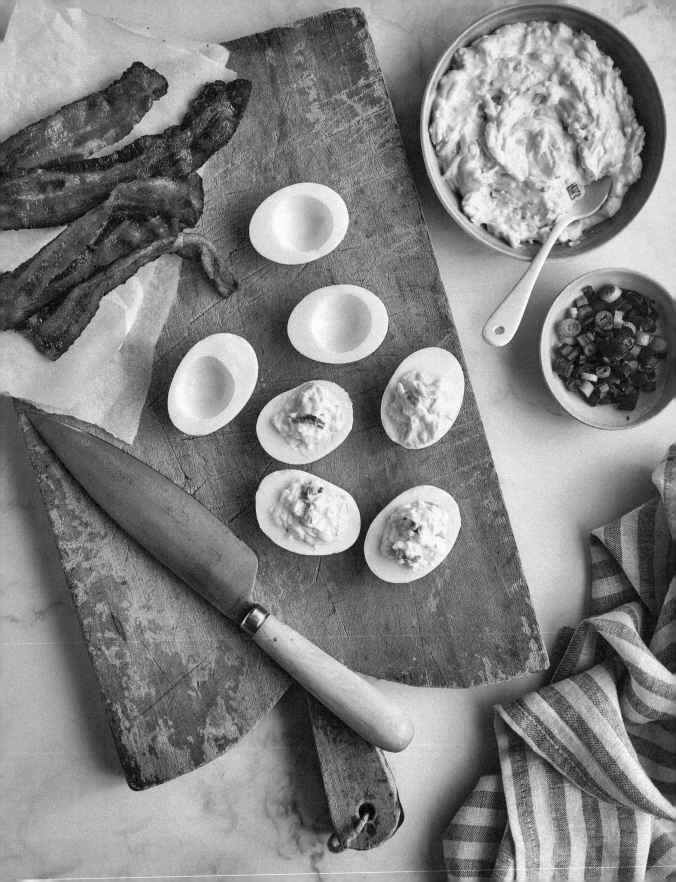

Contents

Loaded Deviled Eggs, page 48

Introduction

Like so many, my journey to better health has been filled with failures, challenges, and triumphs, all of which have guided me to right where I am—where I'm supposed to be. My love of cooking and my passion for the keto lifestyle have led me here, writing a cookbook for people who want a simple approach to the ketogenic diet, and I couldn't be more excited.

Truth be told, we often complicate things with the best intentions. It's the reason people quickly get overwhelmed and quit endeavors before they've even begun. I was introduced to the keto diet at a time in my life when I was desperate to make a change, improve my health, prioritize my well-being, and make a permanent transformation. But my life was busy and chaotic, and I needed a simple approach to this lifestyle to be successful. After years of searching, that's finally what I found.

My love for cooking and amazing food started in my childhood. I've always felt like cooking was a calling, but my relationship with food was a different story. My struggles with health and weight began at 19, when I was diagnosed with polycystic ovarian syndrome (PCOS) and idiopathic intracranial hypertension (IIH), two disorders that are known to cause, or be caused by, weight gain. All of a sudden, I was in a position I had never been in before: I was sick and overweight.

I spent years trying to get these conditions under control with different diets, medications, and exercise, but I was never able to make any significant headway. Finally, one day I received advice about my diet from a doctor that changed my life: "Keep it simple. Eat meat and vegetables." So I did. And I finally began seeing the changes I had waited years to see. Not only did I lose weight, but my symptoms improved with time and my IIH went into remission. My doctors were shocked by my progress, and they encouraged me to continue whatever I was doing. At last, I was in control!

Of course, my weight loss journey was not a linear one. I tried new things here and there, but I always found myself going back to what was easy and worked. I eventually transitioned from a low-carb diet to a keto lifestyle to amplify the health benefits, but the goal has always been to keep it simple. This continues to be my advice for anyone who asks about how to get started on the keto diet or is struggling on their journey.

No matter what your past diet experience or what your health goals may be, you too can reap the benefits of the keto diet and make it work for you by using the straightforward guidelines and helpful tips that follow and by cooking and enjoying the simple recipes in this book. They use fresh, easy-to-find ingredients and common cooking methods. And keto cooking has never been more delicious! I sincerely hope this book helps you find a keto regimen that fits with your life-style—one that is full of easy, satisfying meals.

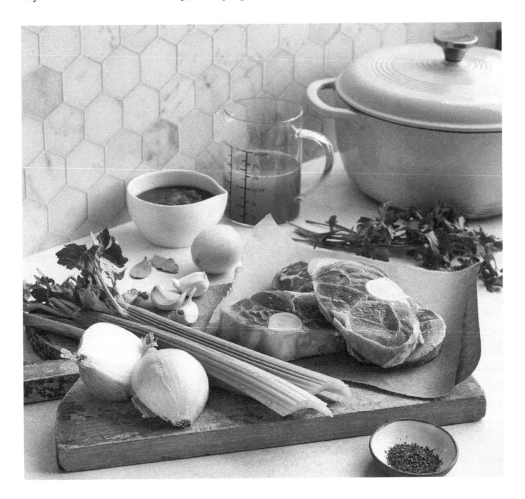

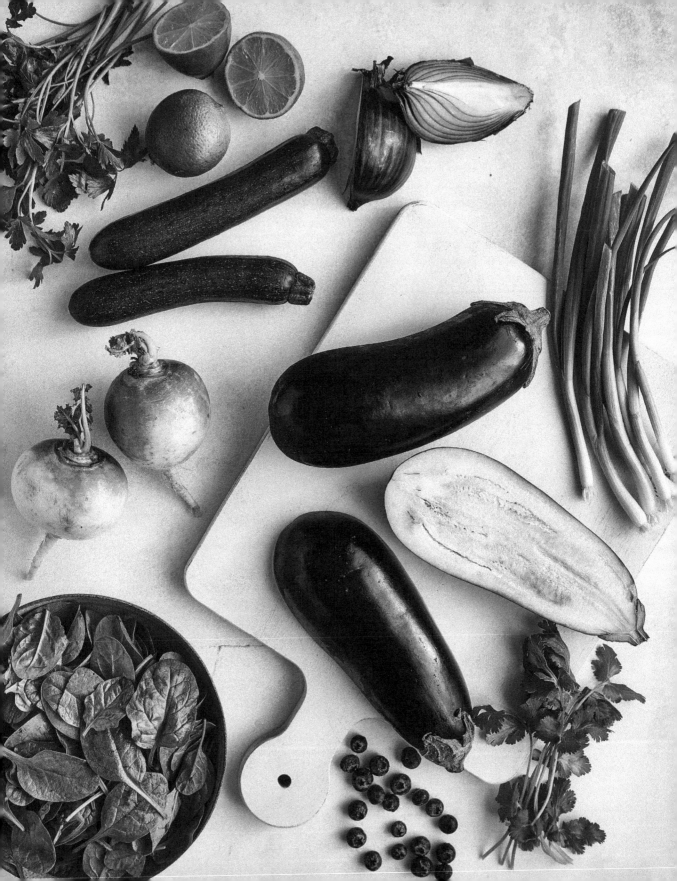

CHAPTER 1

The Simple Guide to Keto Success

Before we get to the good stuff and jump into the kitchen, it's important to understand some essential information about the keto diet. That includes the benefits of this lifestyle, how to get started, why the diet works, and a few tips and tidbits to help you proceed on your journey to better health. Let's get to it!

Making the Keto Diet Work with Your Lifestyle

Chances are if you picked up this book, you're looking to make positive changes to your lifestyle to improve your health. Let me be the first to commend you and say how proud I am of you for taking this first step. It takes courage to make a lifestyle change, and while it can be challenging, you and your health are worth the effort.

Although many people begin the keto diet for weight loss, they often quickly realize there are additional benefits—most notably increased energy and mental clarity, improvement in blood glucose and other health markers, decreased inflammation, and much more. The best part is that you can enjoy these benefits without feeling deprived or constantly hungry. You're free to enjoy the foods you love, like bacon, steak, and cheese, without counting every calorie. In fact, once you understand the nutritional guidelines of the keto diet, it's easy to set achievable goals and develop a plan you can stick with, whether you're looking to lose weight, improve other health issues, or simply stay in shape.

The key to success in the beginning of your keto journey is simplicity. One of the biggest mistakes people make is quickly becoming overwhelmed by mountains of information and getting frustrated by wrestling with complicated recipes and unfamiliar ingredients. The good news is it doesn't have to be this way. The keto diet can easily be adapted to fit your lifestyle, and amazing keto recipes don't have to be complex. This book is full of delicious, simple, straightforward keto recipes that will satisfy nearly every craving and suit any occasion.

Committing to something new or making a change can be exciting, but it can also be intimidating if you don't lay the proper groundwork. That being said, it's important to understand what happens in your body when you eat a keto diet and why this lifestyle works for so many.

Why the Keto Diet Works

There are entire books dedicated to explaining the science behind the keto diet, but to be successful, you just need to know the basics of what happens to your body when you're in ketosis and how the foods you eat affect your efforts.

A proper ketogenic diet is a high-fat, moderate-protein, and very low-carbohydrate way of eating that causes your body to use fat for fuel instead of carbs. More specifically, when you're eating a traditional high-carb diet, your body creates glucose from the carbohydrates you eat and then burns glucose for energy. When carbs are removed and the body no longer has a carb source to make glucose, it switches to another type of fuel, using what it has access to—dietary and body fat. This fat is used to make ketones, which the body uses as an alternative source of fuel. When your body is being fueled by ketones, it's said to be in a state of ketosis.

So now you know what it means to be in ketosis, but how do you know what exactly to eat? Well, if you've researched the keto diet, you've probably heard of "macros," which is short for macronutrients and refers to protein, fat, and carbohydrates. Each type of macronutrient provides a certain amount of energy per gram, and you need the right combination, or macro ratio, to help ensure your body enters a state of ketosis and maintains it while getting all the nutrition you need to thrive. Macros are typically shown as percentages of your daily calories.

Speaking of calories, it's important to note that everyone's optimal caloric intake is different and depends on a number of factors, including metabolism, body composition, and exercise regime, among other factors.

Just as your optimal caloric intake is unique, your macro ratio will more than likely need to be adjusted at some point to achieve the results you want. An average person on a ketogenic diet will get 20 to 25 percent of their calories from protein, 70 to 75 percent from fats, and 5 percent or less from carbohydrates. However, it's important to understand that macros are used as a guideline and are not set in stone.

Calculating macros can be confusing for some, but it doesn't have to be. For help calculating your macros in grams, use a calculator like the one at ruled.me to get a solid place to start. Some people find it useful to log meals and track macros with an app, especially in the beginning. All the recipes in this book contain macro percentages and nutritional information and have a net carb count of 6 grams or less to help you stay on track. (See page 10 for more on net carbs and total carbs.)

Once you've calculated your macros, you'll have a daily protein goal and a certain amount of fat to use to help with hunger. Typically, daily carbs are limited to 20 grams, but this can vary depending on the individual.

Your individual macro ratio allows for quite a bit of variety in terms of what you can eat at every meal. Stocking your kitchen with a wide assortment of keto-friendly ingredients is a great first step.

5 Easy Steps to Help You Get Started on the Keto Diet

Starting a keto diet does require some lifestyle changes, but it doesn't have to be overwhelming. Here are a few tidbits I learned on my own keto journey that made the transition much easier.

1. **Avoid temptation.** Give away or donate non-keto foods and ingredients. Removing temptation will make it easier to stick to your plan and reach your goals.

2. **Have a goal in mind.** It's likely you have a vision for what you're hoping to accomplish while living a keto lifestyle, why it's important, and what it will mean for you to achieve your goal. Focusing on your goal and your "why" is powerful motivation and provides a path for you to track progress and ensure you're headed in the right direction.

3. **Calculate and track your macros.** Once you have a goal in mind, it's important to put together a plan for how you'll get there. Use a macro calculator like the one at ruled.me to calculate your daily macros, and use an app like MyFitnessPal or Carb Manager to track meals and macros. This creates a valuable guide to help you make adjustments to your diet along the way to get the results you want.

4. **Plan your daily meals in advance.** In the morning, log everything you plan to eat for the day into your food tracker and adjust your food or portions accordingly to meet your protein goal and ensure you're under your carb limit for the day. This way, every day is a win!

5. **Be prepared.** Keep keto-friendly foods prepared and on hand for quick meals and snacks when cravings hit. Pack a keto-friendly snack in your bag or desk for emergency cravings and surprise situations.

How to Tell If You're in Ketosis

When you first begin a keto diet, it's important to monitor your ketone levels so you're able to truly know if you're in ketosis. Most people should start noticing signs of ketosis within three to four days of beginning the diet. Keep in mind that factors such as stress and sleep can also affect ketosis. The following are signs and symptoms you may experience that suggest you're in ketosis.

» **Fruity or sweet-smelling breath**

» **Dry mouth or increased thirst**

» **Frequent urination**

» **Weight loss**

» **Appetite suppression**

» **Increased mental clarity and energy**

» **Positive ketone test**

Although your body will give you signs, there are three ways to know without a doubt that you're in ketosis: urine ketone strips, breath monitoring, or blood ketone testing. I prefer blood ketone testing over the others due to ease, accuracy, and reliability. Blood ketone testing is the most accurate way to measure ketones and requires only a finger prick and a drop of blood. The goal is a blood ketone level of 0.5 mmol/L or higher. Just keep in mind that while the monitors are affordable, the test strips they use are expensive. If you're interested in purchasing a ketone meter, I recommend checking out Keto-Mojo.

Knowing you're in ketosis not only confirms your body is burning fat, but also acts as motivation to stay on track and shows you that your hard work is paying off.

Keto Kitchen Essentials

The key to a smooth transition into the keto lifestyle is being well prepared, so you'll want to have certain ingredients and equipment on hand. Having a refrigerator and pantry stocked with keto staples makes throwing together a simple, delicious meal effortless and enjoyable.

Refrigerator Staples

Here are some common, store-bought fresh ingredients for your refrigerator and freezer that will serve as the backbone for many of the keto recipes found in this book.

Avocado: Loaded with more potassium than bananas, avocados are delicious and packed with healthy fats and fiber. Smash them up into guacamole for a quick dip, dice them for a salad, or use them in a smoothie for a super creamy treat.

Butter: I use salted butter in my recipes unless otherwise noted.

Cream cheese: Use full-fat cream cheese to add creaminess and body to savory dishes like soups and sauces. It's also used in keto baked goods to help create structure.

Eggs: Eggs are perfect for a quick meal and are often used in keto baking to help bind ingredients and add structure to breads and cakes. The recipes here all use large eggs.

Frozen cauliflower rice: With a mild flavor and rice-like texture, this low-carb rice alternative is great to have on hand for a quick side or to add to soups and casseroles.

Heavy (whipping) cream: Use heavy cream to make rich sauces or whip it up and add a dollop to your favorite keto dessert.

Keto-friendly mayonnaise: Homemade (see Three-Minute Mayo, page 178) or store-bought keto mayo is perfect for dips, deviled eggs, or slathering on a lettuce wrap or bunless burger.

Parmesan cheese: Parmesan is great to have on hand for anything from breading chicken tenders or pork chops to topping scrambled eggs or a salad. Grate your own to avoid the starches found in pre-shredded cheese.

Unsweetened almond milk: Plant-based, nondairy, and low-carb, almond milk makes a great substitute for regular milk in recipes. Be sure to use an unflavored and unsweetened almond milk.

Pantry Staples

The recipes in this book rely on a small number of pantry items. Some you will likely already have and others you may need to add to your grocery list.

Almond and coconut flours: Almond and coconut flours are useful to have on hand for keto baking and cooking. Mixed together, they create great texture in keto baked goods and are often used in savory recipes as well.

Avocado oil: Mild in flavor, with a high smoke point, avocado oil is my favorite to use for anything from sautéing and frying to baking and no-cook recipes like salad dressing.

Bone broth: This comes in boxes. Be sure your bone broth has no added sugar and preferably is gluten-free.

Coconut milk and cream: Full-fat coconut milk and cream work nicely in keto cooking and baking as dairy-free alternatives to cream.

Pasta alternatives: Shirataki noodles are made from the konjac plant and are very low in carbs. They do not have much flavor on their own, but they absorb the flavors of whatever they are cooked with. Palmini pasta is made from low-carb hearts of palm. It's hearty and absorbs flavors well, making it great for spaghetti, stroganoff, and even soups. Find your favorite alternative and stock up.

Pork rinds: Sometimes called pork skins, this keto snack is easily transformed into everything from breading to breakfast cereal. Even if you're not a fan of pork rinds themselves, you'll be pleasantly surprised by how delicious they can be when used in recipes.

Sweeteners: Blends of monkfruit and erythritol are tasty, versatile, and easily found in both powdered and granulated forms. I also like to keep allulose (or a sweetener blend that includes allulose) on hand, as I find it works better in some dessert recipes because it acts more like traditional sugar (for example, it will caramelize). All the recipes in this book use sweeteners that measure like sugar in a 1:1 ratio. (I'll refer to them in the recipes as 1:1 sweetener and specify powdered or granulated.) Be aware that some powdered or confectioners'-style sweeteners are twice as sweet as sugar, or 2:1, so if you're using something like that, you will want to reduce the amount of sweetener by half.

Equipment Essentials

While the recipes in this book don't require much in the way of equipment, you will need a large skillet, a saucepan, a few mixing bowls, a good knife and a cutting board, and measuring cups and spoons. There are a few other essentials that will also make your time in the kitchen much easier.

Baking sheets: From baking cookies to cooking an entire meal, 13-by-18-inch baking sheets are a must-have in any kitchen.

Blender or immersion blender: A traditional stand blender or an immersion blender is convenient to have for making quick dressings, mayonnaise, sauces, dips, soups, and more.

Dutch oven or heavy stockpot: It's ideal for cooking soups, stews, and one-pot meals.

Electric mixer: Either a stand mixer or an electric handheld mixer will work well for whipping cream or eggs and mixing ingredients for keto baked goods and desserts.

Waffle iron: One of my favorite kitchen gadgets is my 4-inch waffle maker. It's the perfect size for chaffles (cheesy keto waffles), but any waffle maker will do.

5 Tips for Saving Time and Money on the Keto Diet

The keto diet often gets a bad reputation for being too expensive or time-consuming, but it doesn't have to be that way. Here are some tips on how you can do keto easily, without breaking the bank.

1. **Skip the grass-fed, organic, free-range, pasture-raised labels.** Many people who advocate or live a keto lifestyle suggest buying only organic proteins and veggies. These are certainly the healthiest options, but if you're strapped for cash, this isn't a requirement. Simply buy the best-quality keto ingredients you can comfortably afford.

2. **Skip the prepackaged keto foods.** I'm sure you've seen the increase in "keto" products available, from shakes and snack bars to fat bombs and cookies. These items are not necessary for your success, plus they're expensive and not always keto. Beware of prepackaged keto foods and always read the labels. Or save money and make it yourself.

3. **Use frozen ingredients.** To save time, use keto-friendly frozen vegetables, like cauliflower rice, to shorten prep time. Frozen berries can be bought in bulk and stored for months, saving you time and money.

4. **Shop with a list.** Heading to the store with a list helps me shop quickly and keeps me from overspending by grabbing items that I don't need. Review your meal plan for the week, check to see what you have on hand, and make your list accordingly. Organize it by grocery store sections (dairy, produce, meat, etc.) for even faster, more efficient shopping trips.

5. **Watch for sales and stock up.** I have a local grocery store that does a buy-one-get-one special on meat cuts every week, and I always stock up. Pay attention to your local store ads, spot deals, stock up when you can, and freeze any surplus.

Keto Diet Best Practices

Aside from having simple recipes and a stocked keto kitchen, there are some useful guidelines to follow that will help you stay on track and achieve your goals.

Avoid the "keto flu." One of the symptoms or side effects of ketosis is frequent urination, which means you're shedding excess water. This is a sign that you're doing things right, but it also causes an imbalance in your electrolytes that can result in flu-like symptoms (headaches, fatigue, etc.). This is commonly referred to as the keto flu. Supplement and track your electrolytes (potassium, magnesium, and sodium) from day one to avoid feeling under the weather.

Track total carbs rather than net carbs. While some people have amazing results tracking net carbs (total carbs minus any fiber and sugar alcohols) in the beginning, others like me find that tracking total carbs yields better results. Be aware some types of fiber raise blood sugar and can cause stalls in your weight loss, so if you're tracking net carbs and not getting the results you want, try looking at total carbs instead.

Protein is a goal; fat is a lever. You've figured out your macros and you know to stay under 20 carbs for the day. What about protein and fat? Well, protein repairs your muscles and tissues, so this is a goal that you want to hit every day. Your fat intake will change from day to day, and you don't have to meet your fat macro daily. Instead, use fat like a lever to control hunger. As your body becomes adapted to ketosis, your need for dietary fat will decrease and body fat will be used for energy needs.

Eat only when you're hungry. One of the side effects and benefits of being in ketosis is appetite suppression, and this is something you want to take advantage of. If you're not hungry, your body is doing its job—don't sabotage it. Your traditional idea of meal times may go right out the window.

Be prepared when you're eating out or ordering in. Whether it's a lunch meeting near the office or dinner with friends, you can still keep it keto. Most establishments have an online menu, so take a look in advance and scout for keto-friendly options. If your plate comes with a starch, like potatoes or rice, ask for it to be left off or substitute with a veggie or a salad. Try to plan ahead: If you know you're going to eat Mexican food, for example, and they put chips and salsa on the table, throw some pork rinds or keto chips in your bag to enjoy with the salsa. Don't stress.

If you fall off the wagon, don't give up. The truth of the matter is we all mess up. So you gave in and took a bite of something off-limits? Consider it a setback, not a failure, and embrace the fact that tomorrow is a new day. A slipup can affect your efforts to stay in ketosis, but as long as you continue to eat keto-friendly foods you will quickly be back on track. You only fail when you decide you and your health are not worth the effort—and you are so worth it!

What's in This Book

I'm so excited to share these simple keto recipes with you. As I said, simplicity is key to an easy start on the keto diet. The recipes in this book are designed to be easy to shop for and prepare, and they're perfect for busy weeknights.

To help guide your stress-free meal planning, this book has many recipes that fall into four "easy" categories: 5 Ingredients or Fewer, 30 Minutes or Less, One-Pot, and No-Cook. Just as it sounds, the recipes labeled 5 Ingredients or Fewer can be made with just five ingredients (not including some "freebies" that you'll most likely already have on hand, like salt, pepper, oil or nonstick cooking spray, and water). Likewise, the 30 Minutes or Less recipes can be prepped and cooked in a half hour or less, making them perfect for quick family dinners or even last-minute entertaining. One-Pot dishes can be made entirely in one pan or pot, keeping kitchen mess and cleanup to a minimum, while No-Cook meals are just what they say.

Finally, I'll let you know which recipes are dairy-free and vegetarian or vegan. And all the recipes include nutritional information to make your mealtime decisions even easier.

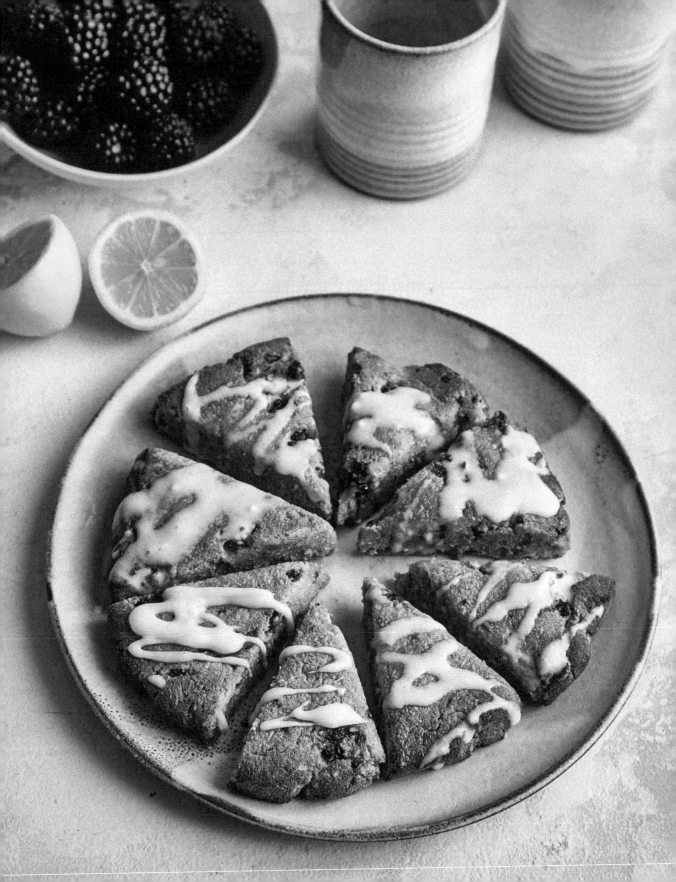

CHAPTER 2

Breakfasts

Blackberry-Lemon Scones, page 19

Triple Berry Cheesecake Smoothie

Prep time: 5 minutes

Quick and easy to make and full of sweet, tangy berry flavor, this keto smoothie has all the deliciousness of a rich, decadent berry cheesecake. It's perfect for a quick breakfast on the go or a refreshing lunch or snack.
Serves 1

½ cup unsweetened almond milk

2 tablespoons avocado

2 tablespoons full-fat cream cheese

1 teaspoon vanilla extract

½ cup frozen strawberry, raspberry, and blackberry blend

2 to 3 tablespoons powdered 1:1 sweetener

Pinch kosher salt

In a high-speed blender, combine the almond milk, avocado, cream cheese, vanilla, berries, sweetener, and salt. Blend on high for 10 to 20 seconds, or until smooth. Pour into a glass and enjoy.

Per Serving Calories 205; Total Fat 16g; Total Carbs 45g; Fiber 4g; Net Carbs 11g; Protein 3g; Macros: Fat 70%/Protein 6%/Carbs 24%

Chocolate-Pecan Smoothie

Prep time: 10 minutes

Creamy, decadent, and incredibly chocolaty this keto shake is perfect for a busy morning, quick lunch, or dessert and reminds me of rocky road ice cream. Thanks to the avocado and pecans, it's also packed with healthy fats and a significant amount of potassium and magnesium, and it's definitely a must-have in your recipe arsenal. **Serves 1**

1⅓ cups unsweetened almond milk

¼ cup raw pecan halves

2 tablespoons avocado

2 tablespoons unsweetened cocoa powder

Pinch kosher salt

2 to 3 tablespoons powdered 1:1 sweetener

3 or 4 ice cubes

In a high-speed blender, combine the almond milk, pecans, avocado, cocoa powder, salt, sweetener, and ice. Blend on high for 10 to 20 seconds, or until smooth. Pour into a glass and enjoy.

Tip: For a different flavor profile, omit the pecans, add 1 tablespoon of no-sugar-added peanut butter, and blend as directed.

Per Serving Calories 309; Total Fat 29g; Total Carbs 47g; Fiber 9g; Net Carbs 8g; Protein 6g; Macros: Fat 84%/ Protein 8%/Carbs 8%

Cinnamon Crunch Cereal

Prep time: 7 minutes Cook time: 10 minutes

Don't be alarmed by the use of pork rinds in this recipe, as they are completely transformed by the cinnamon glaze. This cereal also makes a great snack to keep on hand. Make a triple or quadruple batch to save prep time during the week. Store it at room temperature in a zip-top bag or sealed container. **Serves 3**

2 ounces pork rinds (about 3 cups), broken into pieces

1½ tablespoons salted butter

3½ tablespoons granulated 1:1 sweetener

1 tablespoon water

1 teaspoon ground cinnamon

½ teaspoon vanilla extract

Unsweetened almond milk, for serving

1. Preheat the oven to 325°F. Line a baking sheet with parchment paper.

2. Place the pork rind pieces in a medium bowl and set aside.

3. In a small saucepan, combine the butter, sweetener, and water. Bring the mixture to a rolling boil and cook for 2 to 3 minutes. Remove from the heat and stir in the cinnamon and vanilla. Slowly drizzle the cinnamon mixture over the pork rind pieces and stir well to coat.

4. Spread the coated pork rinds evenly on the prepared baking sheet along with any syrup that has crystalized in the bowl. Bake for 10 to 12 minutes, stirring halfway through and keeping a close eye on the cereal so it doesn't burn.

5. Let the cereal cool completely on the pan. Serve with unsweetened almond milk.

Per Serving Calories: 156; Total Fat: 12g; Total Carbs: 15g; Fiber: 1g; Net Carbs: 1g; Protein: 12g; Macros: Fat 69%/ Protein 30%/Carbs 1%

Orange-Coconut Muffins

Prep time: 10 minutes Cook time: 20 minutes

These easy muffins feature a delicious coconut and orange flavor combo and make a great grab-and-go breakfast. These muffins will keep in the freezer for up to one month. **Makes 10 muffins**

1 cup almond flour

¼ cup coconut flour

2½ teaspoons baking powder

¼ teaspoon kosher salt

6 tablespoons granulated 1:1 sweetener

4 large eggs

1 egg yolk

1 teaspoon vanilla extract

¼ teaspoon coconut extract (optional)

1½ teaspoons grated orange zest

⅓ cup coconut oil, melted and cooled

1½ tablespoons unsweetened shredded coconut

1. Preheat the oven to 350°F. Prepare a standard 12-cup muffin tin with 10 liners.

2. In a small bowl, combine the almond flour, coconut flour, baking powder, salt, and sweetener.

3. Using a stand mixer with a whisk attachment or using a handheld mixer in a large bowl, whip the eggs and yolk until light and foamy, about 2 minutes. Add the vanilla extract, coconut extract (if using), and orange zest to the eggs and stir well. Add the flour mixture and coconut oil to the eggs and mix on medium speed until the ingredients are combined, scraping down the sides at least once.

4. Using a cookie scoop or a large serving spoon, divide the batter among the prepared muffin cups. Sprinkle about ½ teaspoon shredded coconut evenly over top of each muffin.

5. Bake for 15 to 18 minutes, or until golden brown on top. Cool the muffins in the pan for 10 minutes, then transfer to a rack to cool completely.

Per Serving (1 muffin) Calories: 178; Total Fat: 16g; Total Carbs: 12g; Fiber: 2g; Net Carbs: 5g; Protein: 5g; Macros: Fat 81%/Protein 11%/Carbs 8%

Coconut Flour Pancakes

Prep time: 10 minutes Cook time: 5 minutes per batch

These are hands down my all-time favorite keto pancakes. This simple recipe comes together in just a few minutes with ingredients you already have in your pantry, and the pancakes are great reheated, making them ideal for weekly meal prep. Serve warm, topped with butter and your favorite sugar-free syrup or with Berry Compote (page 20).

Makes 9 small pancakes

4 eggs, beaten

⅓ cup coconut flour

1¼ teaspoons baking powder

Pinch kosher salt

¼ cup unsweetened almond milk

1 teaspoon vanilla extract

2 tablespoons granulated 1:1 sweetener

3 tablespoons butter, melted, plus more for serving

Coconut oil spray or nonstick cooking spray

1. In a medium bowl, combine the eggs, coconut flour, baking powder, salt, almond milk, vanilla, sweetener, and butter and stir until well combined.

2. Coat a griddle pan lightly with coconut oil spray and preheat over medium-low heat.

3. Pour ¼ cup of batter onto the griddle for each pancake, spreading the batter slightly. Cook for 2 to 3 minutes, or until the bottoms are golden brown. Using a spatula, carefully flip the pancakes and cook for another 1 to 2 minutes on the other side. Repeat until all the batter is used up.

Tip: Keto pancakes are often a little more fragile due to the lack of gluten holding things together. A thin metal spatula or slotted turner, sometimes called a fish spatula, makes the perfect pancake flip a breeze.

Per Serving (1 pancake) Calories: 83; Total Fat: 7g; Total Carbs: 5g; Fiber: 2g; Net Carbs: 1g; Protein: 3g; Macros: Fat 76%/Protein 14%/Carbs 10%

Blackberry-Lemon Scones

Prep time: 10 minutes Cook time: 15 minutes

These flavor-packed scones are my family's favorite keto breakfast. Black-berries are one of the lowest-carb fruits, making them the perfect fruity addition to these lemony scones. Chopping up the blackberries ensures that every bite of these breakfast treats has a burst of berry flavor.

Makes 8 scones

1¼ cups almond flour

3 tablespoons coconut flour

2 teaspoons baking powder

¼ teaspoon kosher salt

2 tablespoons granulated 1:1 sweetener, divided

¼ teaspoon ground cinnamon

1 teaspoon grated lemon zest

1 egg, beaten

2 tablespoons sour cream

1⅛ teaspoons vanilla extract, divided

2 tablespoons butter, melted

⅓ cup blackberries, coarsely chopped

2 tablespoons powdered 1:1 sweetener

1 tablespoon heavy (whipping) cream

1. Preheat the oven to 375°F. Line a large baking sheet with parchment paper.

2. In a medium bowl, combine the almond flour, coconut flour, baking powder, salt, granulated sweetener, cinnamon, and lemon zest.

3. In another bowl, whisk together the egg, sour cream, 1 teaspoon vanilla, and butter. Add the dry ingredients to the egg mixture and stir well to combine. Gently fold in the chopped blackberries.

4. Scoop the dough into 8 mounds and place on the baking sheet. Pat each mound of dough into a circle about ½ inch thick. Bake for 12 to 15 minutes, or until the edges are golden brown.

5. To make the glaze, in a small bowl, combine the powdered sweetener and the remaining ⅛ teaspoon vanilla with the heavy cream and mix until smooth. Drizzle the glaze over the warm scones and serve.

Per Serving (1 scone) Calories: 162; Total Fat: 14g; Total Carbs: 13g; Fiber: 3g; Net Carbs: 7g; Protein: 5g; Macros: Fat 78%/Protein 12%/Carbs 10%

Chaffles with Berry Compote and Whipped Mascarpone Cream

Prep time: 12 minutes Cook time: 5 minutes per chaffle

Chaffles are keto-friendly waffles made with an egg-and-cheese-based batter. It may sound weird, but trust me, they're delish! These lightly sweetened vanilla chaffles are perfect when you're craving something sweet and fruity to start your day. This recipe makes eight chaffles, which is just right for a hungry family, or you can store leftover chaffles in the refrigerator for up to 4 days for a quick weekday breakfast. They can be reheated in a toaster, air fryer, oven, or the waffle maker. **Serves 8**

FOR THE BERRY COMPOTE

½ cup raspberries, divided

½ cup blackberries, divided

½ cup quartered strawberries, divided

1 to 2 tablespoons granulated 1:1 sweetener

¼ teaspoon vanilla extract

FOR THE MASCARPONE CREAM

¾ cup heavy (whipping) cream

1 to 2 tablespoons powdered 1:1 sweetener

½ teaspoon vanilla extract

⅓ cup mascarpone cheese, at room temperature

TO MAKE THE BERRY COMPOTE

1. Place ¼ cup each raspberries, blackberries, and strawberries in a large bowl. Set aside.

2. In a blender, blend the remaining berries, granulated sweetener, and vanilla on high until smooth. Pour over the remaining berries and chill until you're ready to use.

TO MAKE THE MASCARPONE CREAM

3. Using a handheld mixer in a large bowl, whip the heavy cream with the powdered sweetener and vanilla until soft peaks form. Add the mascarpone cheese and continue whipping on high until stiff peaks form. This should take less than a minute.

4. Cover and chill until you're ready to use.

FOR THE CHAFFLES

¼ cup cream cheese, at room temperature

2 eggs

¾ cup shredded mozzarella cheese

½ teaspoon vanilla extract

¼ teaspoon baking powder

3 teaspoons granulated 1:1 sweetener

¼ cup almond flour

TO MAKE THE CHAFFLES

5. Preheat the waffle iron.

6. In a large bowl, combine the cream cheese, eggs, mozzarella cheese, vanilla, baking powder, sweetener, and almond flour and stir until well combined.

7. Once the waffle iron is hot, place about 2 tablespoons of batter in the center of the waffle maker and close. Cook until browned and steam is no longer coming out of the waffle maker, 3 to 5 minutes.

8. Remove the chaffle from the waffle iron and cool on a wire rack. Repeat step 7 until all the batter is used up.

9. To serve, place a chaffle on a plate and top with about 3 tablespoons of mascarpone cream and 2 tablespoons of berry compote.

Tip: Don't use pre-shredded mozzarella cheese; shred it yourself. Pre-shredded cheese is tossed with starch to keep it from sticking together, so the cheese doesn't melt as well when you're cooking.

Per Serving Calories: 224; Total Fat: 21g; Total Carbs: 10g; Fiber: 2g; Net Carbs: 3g; Protein: 6g; Macros: Fat 84%/ Protein 11%/Carbs 5%

Fat Head Bagels with Blackberry Cream Cheese

Prep time: 15 minutes Cook time: 20 minutes

Bagels, like other carb-heavy foods, are something you might miss after going keto. Thankfully, there is fat head dough, a gluten-free dough replacement (named after Tom Naughton's documentary *Fat Head*) made from cheese and almond flour which is used to make these tasty bagels.
Makes 8 bagels

3½ cups shredded mozzarella cheese

1½ cups almond flour

2 tablespoons cream cheese, plus ½ cup

1 teaspoon kosher salt, plus a pinch

⅓ cup blackberries

1 teaspoon freshly squeezed lemon juice

1. Preheat the oven to 350°F. Line a baking sheet with parchment paper.

2. In a medium microwave-safe bowl, mix together the mozzarella cheese and almond flour. Add 2 tablespoons cream cheese on top and microwave on high for 2 minutes. Stir the mixture and microwave again for 1 minute.

3. Stir in the salt until the mixture forms a dough ball. Divide the dough into 8 equal pieces. Roll each piece into a log, then form each log into a circle, pinching the ends together to make a bagel shape.

4. Place the bagels on the baking sheet and bake for about 18 minutes, or until the bottoms begin to brown and become firm. Remove from the oven and let cool on the baking sheet for about 5 minutes.

5. Make the blackberry cream cheese. Using a handheld mixer (or by hand) in a medium bowl, combine ½ cup cream cheese, the blackberries, lemon juice, and a pinch salt and beat until well combined. Spread the blackberry cream cheese on the bagels.

Tip: Use mozzarella cheese with a higher fat content to get a better dough texture.

Per Serving (1 bagel with cream cheese) Calories: 343; Total Fat: 29g; Total Carbs: 7g; Fiber: 3g; Net Carbs: 4g; Protein: 16g; Macros: Fat 76%/Protein 19%/Carbs 5%

Granola Bars

Prep time: 10 minutes Cook time: 20 minutes

These grab-and-go breakfast bars taste like a treat, but with protein-rich hazelnuts, almonds, and peanut butter, healthy fats, and plenty of antioxidants, they are just the thing to start your morning off right. Make an extra batch to enjoy as snacks throughout the week or on long car rides. Refrigerate them in an airtight container for up to 2 weeks. **Makes 12 bars**

1 cup almonds

1 cup hazelnuts

1 cup unsweetened coconut flakes

1 egg

¼ cup coconut oil, melted

¼ cup unsweetened peanut butter

½ cup dark chocolate chips

1 tablespoon vanilla extract

1 tablespoon ground cinnamon

Pinch kosher salt

1. Preheat the oven to 350°F.

2. In a food processor, pulse together the almonds and hazelnuts for 1 to 2 minutes, or until roughly chopped. You want them pretty fine but not turning into nut butter. Transfer them to a large bowl.

3. Add the coconut flakes, egg, coconut oil, peanut butter, chocolate chips, vanilla, cinnamon, and salt and stir well. Transfer the mixture to an 8- or 9-inch square baking dish and gently press into an even layer. Bake for 15 to 20 minutes, or until golden brown. Let cool and cut into 12 bars.

Tip: Add 2 tablespoons of unsweetened cocoa powder to the bar mix before baking. Or if you have room for extra carbs and want to add some fruit, stir in ½ cup of chopped fresh raspberries.

Per Serving (1 bar) Calories: 321; Total Fat: 29g; Total Carbs: 11g; Fiber: 5g; Net Carbs: 6g; Protein: 7g; Macros: Fat 81%/Protein 9%/Carbs 10%

Smoked Turkey, Bacon, and Avocado Breakfast Salad

Prep time: 10 minutes

Can't decide between breakfast and lunch? This breakfast salad is loaded with fiber, protein, and healthy fats to jump-start your day—no matter when it starts. I came up with this salad years ago when traditional breakfast food never seemed to interest me. To keep things quick and easy, pick up a quality smoked turkey from the deli counter—skip the prepackaged lunch meat that contains sugar and additives. **Serves 2**

1 small head romaine lettuce, chopped

⅓ cup shredded Monterey Jack cheese

1 cup smoked turkey deli meat, cut into strips

2 bacon slices, cooked until crispy and crumbled

½ cup halved grape tomatoes

½ avocado, peeled and diced

2 eggs, poached (page 34) or fried

Your favorite salad dressing, for topping

1. In a large bowl, toss together the lettuce, Monterey Jack cheese, turkey, bacon, tomatoes and avocado.

2. Divide into two servings. Top each with an egg and dress with your favorite salad dressing.

Tip: If you're a fan of poached eggs, make a few in advance and keep them in the refrigerator. After the eggs have finished poaching, place them in ice water and store them in the refrigerator for up to 4 days. To reheat, dip them in hot water for 20 to 30 seconds.

Per Serving Calories: 420; Total Fat: 26g; Total Carbs: 21g; Fiber: 9g; Net Carbs: 12g; Protein: 29g; Macros: Fat 56%/ Protein 28%/Carbs 16%

Broccoli Quiche

Prep time: 10 minutes Cook time: 30 minutes

Quiche traditionally has a thick crust and combines eggs with various fillings. In this crustless keto version, broccoli takes center stage, with yogurt and cheese providing complementary tanginess. It's a filling breakfast that's easy to make ahead of time for busy mornings. **Serves 2**

Nonstick cooking spray

1 egg

5 egg whites

½ cup plain nonfat
Greek yogurt

1 teaspoon kosher salt

¼ teaspoon freshly ground
black pepper

1 tablespoon minced garlic

1 cup broccoli florets

1 cup shredded
cheddar cheese

1. Preheat the oven to 400°F. Spray a 9-inch pie pan with nonstick cooking spray.

2. In a medium bowl, mix together the egg, egg whites, yogurt, salt, pepper, and garlic. Fold in the broccoli and cheddar cheese.

3. Pour the mixture into the prepared pie pan and bake for 30 minutes, or until the eggs are set. Remove the quiche from the oven and let cool for a few minutes before serving.

Tip: This quiche will be thin, so don't wait for it to puff up. Think of it more as a broccoli crêpe that you could even roll up to eat.

Per Serving Calories: 360; Total Fat: 22g; Total Carbs: 9g; Fiber: 1g; Net Carbs: 8g; Protein: 31g; Macros: Fat 55%/ Protein 34%/Carbs 11%

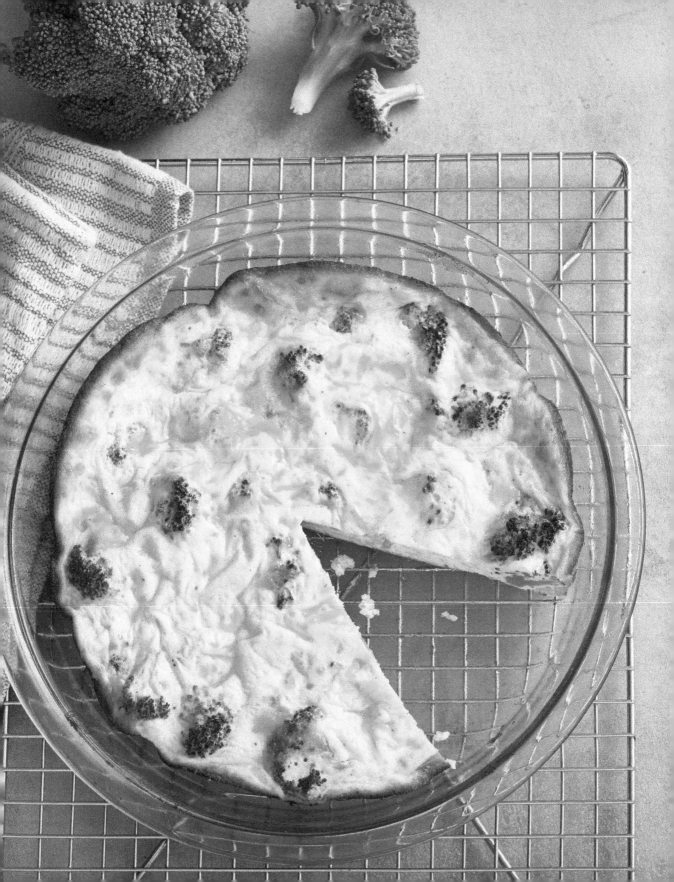

Chicken Fajita Frittata

Prep time: 10 minutes Cook time: 35 minutes

I'll admit it, I'm a frittata fanatic. They're not only perfect for keto, but they quickly come together in one skillet; they're great for breakfast, lunch, or dinner; and they're incredibly delicious. This frittata is full of Tex-Mex flair with spiced-up chicken, sautéed peppers and onions, and creamy Monterey Jack cheese. Serve topped with avocado and a dollop of sour cream. One bite will make you a frittata fanatic, too. **Serves 6**

10 eggs

¼ cup sour cream

¼ cup heavy
(whipping) cream

½ teaspoon freshly ground
black pepper, divided

1½ teaspoons kosher
salt, divided

1½ cups shredded Monterey
Jack cheese, divided

2 tablespoons butter

1 pound boneless,
skinless chicken thighs
(about 4 thighs), cut into
1-inch pieces

½ teaspoon garlic powder

½ teaspoon ground cumin

½ medium yellow
onion, sliced

1 green bell pepper, seeded
and cut into strips

1. Preheat the oven to 350°F.

2. In a large bowl, put the eggs, sour cream, heavy cream, ¼ teaspoon black pepper, and ½ teaspoon salt. Gently whisk to combine but don't whip. Gently stir in 1 cup cheese and set aside.

3. Preheat a medium nonstick oven-safe skillet over medium-high heat and melt the butter. Add the chicken and season with the remaining 1 teaspoon salt, remaining ¼ teaspoon black pepper, garlic powder, and cumin. Cook over medium-high heat for about 5 minutes. Reduce the heat to medium, add the onion and bell pepper, and continue to cook until the onions are translucent and begin to caramelize and the chicken is golden and cooked through, 4 to 5 minutes.

4. Reduce the heat to medium-low and spread the chicken and veggie mixture evenly across the bottom of the skillet. Give the egg mixture a final gentle stir and pour evenly over the chicken-veggie mixture. Move the chicken mixture around a little so the eggs can get down to the bottom of the skillet. Sprinkle the remaining ½ cup cheese evenly over the top but don't stir.

5. Place the pan in the oven and bake for 20 to 25 minutes, or until the eggs are set and cooked and the center still has a little jiggle. Carefully remove from the oven and cool for at least 5 to 10 minutes. Serve warm or at room temperature.

Tip: To get this frittata on the table in no time flat, use any leftover cooked chicken you have in the refrigerator from weeknight meals.

Per Serving Calories: 404; Total Fat: 30g; Total Carbs: 4g; Fiber: 1g; Net Carbs: 3g; Protein: 29g; Macros: Fat 67%/ Protein 29%/Carbs 4%

Sausage, Egg, and Radish Hash

Prep time: 10 minutes Cook time: 45 minutes

Everyone loves a breakfast skillet. Most contain potatoes, though, which are not on the keto food list. This version uses radishes instead. If you've never had sautéed radishes for breakfast, you will be pleasantly surprised because the flavor is incredible. You have the option of using ghee or butter in this recipe. Ghee is clarified butter, meaning its water and milk solids are removed, leaving a higher concentration of fat compared to butter. **Serves 2**

6 bacon slices

5 ounces breakfast sausage patties

1 teaspoon ghee or unsalted butter

12 small radishes, diced

½ teaspoon kosher salt

¼ teaspoon freshly ground black pepper

½ onion, diced

1 bell pepper, any color, seeded and diced

4 eggs

¼ cup shredded mozzarella cheese

1. Preheat the oven to 400°F. Line a large baking sheet with aluminum foil.

2. Lay the bacon on one half of the baking sheet in a single layer and place the sausage patties on the other half. Bake for 20 minutes, then transfer the meats to a paper towel–lined plate to drain. Dice the bacon and sausage and set aside.

3. In a cast-iron skillet or sauté pan, heat the ghee over medium-high heat. Add the radishes and cook until they begin to brown and soften, stirring occasionally, about 10 minutes. Season with salt and black pepper. Add the onion and bell pepper and cook until they are soft, about 5 minutes. Reduce the heat to medium and add the cooked bacon and sausage and stir to heat through, about 5 minutes.

4. In a small sauté pan, cook the eggs to your liking.

5. Top the hash and meat in the skillet with the mozzarella cheese and cook until melted, about 5 minutes. Top the hash with the eggs and serve.

Tip: If you don't have breakfast sausage, you can also use ham, a vegetable, or more bacon.

Per Serving Calories: 624; Total Fat: 51g; Total Carbs: 10g; Fiber: 2g; Net Carbs: 8g; Protein: 32g; Macros: Fat 74%/ Protein 21%/Carbs 5%

Bacon-Cheddar-Chive Scones

Prep time: 10 minutes Cook time: 30 minutes

If the words "bacon" and "cheddar" didn't grab your attention, perhaps the fact that these scones are also light and fluffy will. Savory scones are just as delicious as their sweet counterparts. They are also low in carbs and super easy to make. You can freeze the leftovers for up to 3 weeks.
Makes 10 scones

4 tablespoons (½ stick) unsalted butter, melted and cooled, plus 1 tablespoon for greasing

½ cup full-fat sour cream

3 eggs, at room temperature

1½ cups almond flour, sifted

½ cup coconut flour

1½ teaspoons baking powder

½ teaspoon kosher salt

4 tablespoons shredded cheddar cheese, divided

4 bacon slices, cooked and crumbled

2 tablespoons chopped fresh chives

1. Preheat the oven to 375°F. Grease a 9-inch oven-safe skillet with 1 tablespoon butter.

2. Using a handheld mixer in a large bowl, combine the remaining 4 tablespoons butter, sour cream, and eggs. Fold in the almond flour, coconut flour, baking powder, and salt using a silicone spatula until fully combined. Then fold in 2 tablespoons cheddar cheese and half of the cooked crumbled bacon.

3. Spread the batter in the skillet. Sprinkle the remaining 2 tablespoons cheese, remaining bacon, and chives on top.

4. Bake for 25 to 30 minutes, or until a toothpick inserted into the center comes out clean. Let cool completely in the skillet, then cut into wedges to serve.

Tip: If you don't have the right size oven-safe skillet, you can use a greased 9-inch round cake pan.

Per Serving (1 scone) Calories: 231; Total Fat: 20g; Total Carbs: 8g; Fiber: 4g; Net Carbs: 4g; Protein: 8g; Macros: Fat 78%/Protein 14%/Carbs 8%

Bacon-Avocado Benedict

Prep time: 15 minutes Cook time: 35 minutes

For years, I only enjoyed eggs Benedict when going out for breakfast. Who knew making a delicious keto version at home would be so easy? This version uses a bacon and chive chaffle in place of the traditional English muffin, topped with creamy avocado and a luscious runny poached egg and drizzled with an easy hollandaise sauce. It's a breakfast that's worthy of five stars. **Serves 4**

2 tablespoons cream cheese, at room temperature

5 eggs, divided

½ cup shredded mozzarella cheese

¼ teaspoon baking powder

2 tablespoons almond flour

3 bacon slices, cooked until crispy and crumbled

2 medium avocados, thinly sliced

Blender Hollandaise (page 179)

1 scallion, both white and green parts, sliced

1. Preheat the waffle iron.

2. In a medium bowl, mix together the cream cheese, 1 egg, mozzarella cheese, baking powder, and almond flour until well combined. Stir in the crumbled bacon.

3. When the waffle iron is hot, place about 2 tablespoons of batter in the center of the waffle maker and close it. Cook until browned and the steam is no longer coming out from the waffle maker, 3 to 5 minutes. Remove the chaffle from the waffle iron and cool on a wire rack. Repeat until all the batter is used up.

continued >

4. Meanwhile, poach the eggs. Add about 4 inches of water to a medium saucepan and bring the water to a boil. Reduce the heat to low. Break 1 egg into a small dish. Using a spoon, swirl the simmering water in a clockwise motion to create a whirlpool. While the water is swirling, gently slip the egg into the center. Poach for 3 to 4 minutes, or until the white is set and the yolk is still runny or done as desired. Remove the egg from the water with a slotted spoon and place on a paper towel–lined plate to drain. Repeat with the remaining 3 eggs.

5. To serve, place a chaffle on each plate and top with some sliced avocado and a poached egg. Top with the hollandaise sauce and scallions.

Tip: One of the trickiest things about poaching eggs is keeping the whites together. To make this easier in the beginning, slip a slotted spoon or a spider skimmer under the egg to gently cradle it in the simmering water while it cooks. This will keep the whites together and gently shape the poached egg.

Per Serving (including sauce) Calories: 563; Total Fat: 53g; Total Carbs: 9g; Fiber: 5g; Net Carbs: 4g; Protein: 17g; Macros: Fat 85%/Protein 12%/Carbs 3%

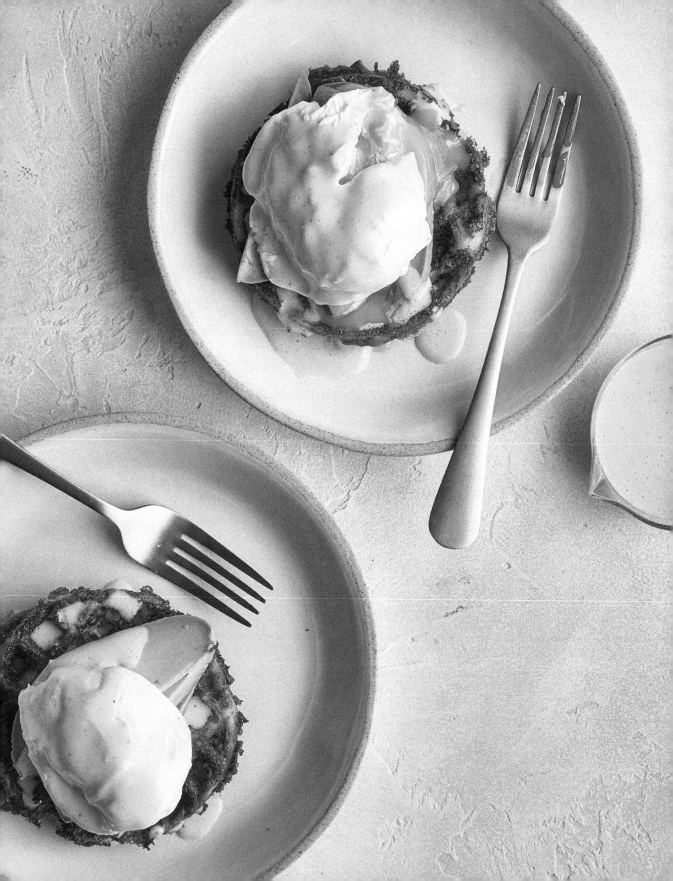

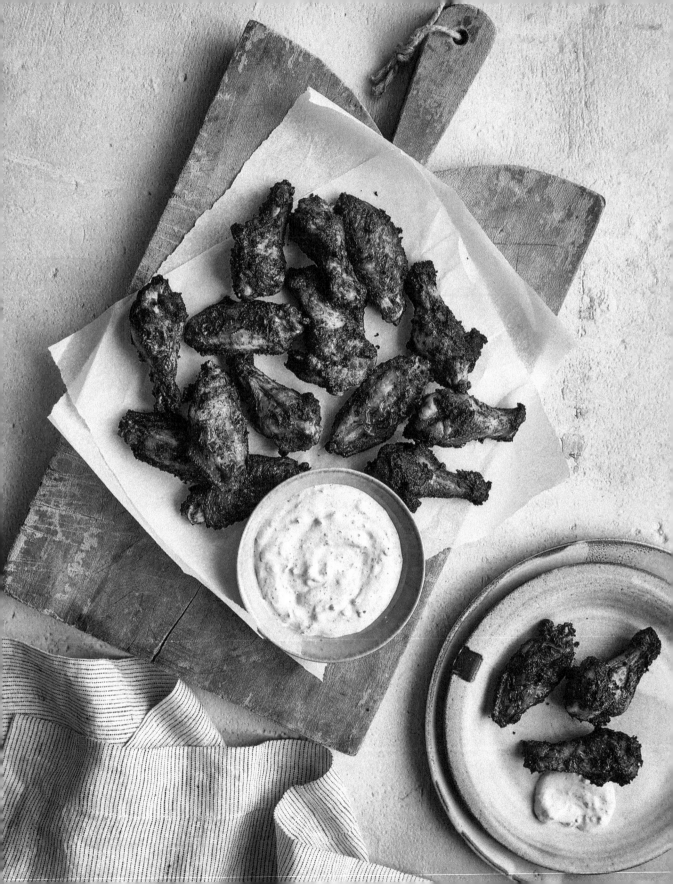

CHAPTER 3

Snacks and Appetizers

Pickle-Brined Chicken Wings, page 47

Sweet and Spicy Pecans

Prep time: 10 minutes Cook time: 20 minutes

Pecans are loaded with vitamins, minerals, and antioxidants. They're also low in carbs, which makes them a great keto-friendly choice. These sweet and spicy pecans are great to have on hand for a quick snack, to add to a salad, or to sprinkle on top of keto vanilla ice cream for a treat. But with nuts, it's easy to eat too many, so be mindful of macros when you're enjoying them. **Serves 8**

2 cups pecan halves

½ teaspoon kosher salt

¾ teaspoon chili powder

¾ teaspoon paprika

¼ teaspoon cayenne pepper

2 tablespoons butter

¼ cup granulated 1:1 sweetener

2 tablespoons water

1. Preheat the oven to 300°F. Line a baking sheet with parchment paper.

2. Place the pecans in a medium bowl and set aside.

3. In a small bowl, combine the salt, chili powder, paprika, and cayenne pepper.

4. In a small saucepan, combine the butter, sweetener, and water. Bring the mixture to a rolling boil and cook for 1 minute. Remove the saucepan from the heat and stir in the spices.

5. Pour the spice mixture over the pecans and stir well to coat. Spread the coated pecans in a single layer on the prepared pan. Bake for 10 minutes, stir, then bake for an additional 7 to 10 minutes. Keep an eye on the pecans toward the end of the cooking time to avoid burning.

6. Cool completely before packing in an airtight container.

Per Serving (¼ cup) Calories: 215; Total Fat: 22g; Total Carbs: 10g; Fiber: 3g; Net Carbs: 4g; Protein: 3g; Macros: Fat 92%/Protein 6%/Carbs 2%

Creamy Avocado Salsa Verde Dip

Prep time: 10 minutes

This addictive, spicy avocado dip is inspired by a dish at one of my favorite Tex-Mex restaurants. Serve it with keto tortilla chips or use it as a dip for veggies or keto crackers, as a dressing on salads, or as a spread on lettuce wraps and burgers—the options are endless. Adjust the heat by choosing a tomatillo salsa with your preferred spice level. **Makes 3 cups**

2 ripe avocados, peeled and pitted (about 1 cup)

4 ounces cream cheese, at room temperature

1 cup sour cream

⅓ cup tomatillo salsa

1 garlic clove, peeled

1 teaspoon kosher salt

½ teaspoon ground cumin

1 bunch cilantro

1 tablespoon freshly squeezed lime juice

In a blender or food processor, blend the avocados, cream cheese, sour cream, tomatillo salsa, garlic, salt, cumin, cilantro and lime juice until smooth and creamy.

Per Serving (1 tablespoon) Calories: 28; Total Fat: 3g; Total Carbs: 1g; Fiber: <1g; Net Carbs: <1g; Protein: <1g; Macros: Fat 96%/Protein 2%/Carbs 2%

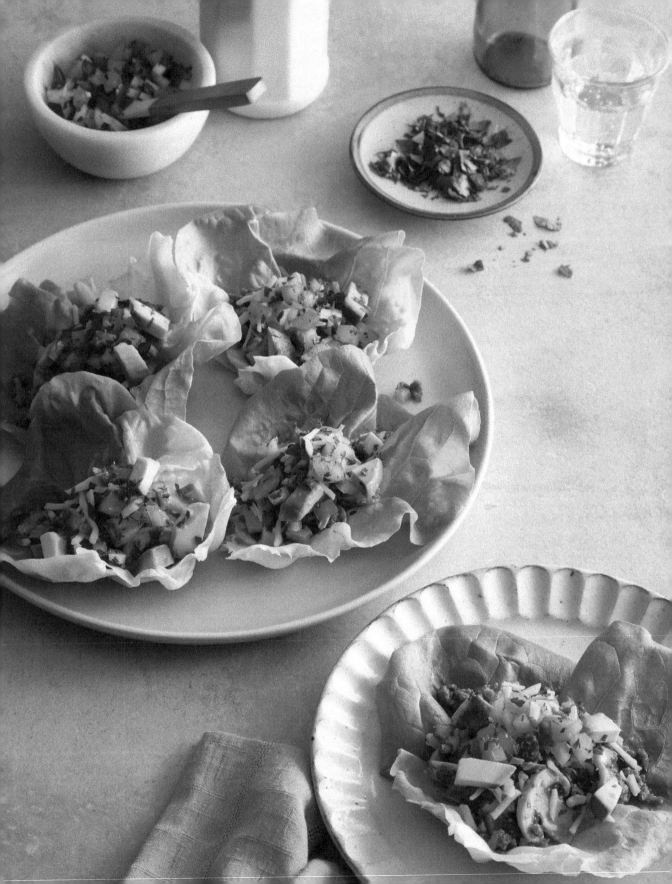

Taco Lettuce Cups

Prep time: 10 minutes Cook time: 10 minutes

Meat substitutes have come a long way in the past few years. If you are new to meat substitutes, these tacos are a great way to learn about them. Most soy-based products are made with GMO soy, so carefully read the package labels before you buy. Boca is a non-GMO brand, which makes it a good choice for these tasty tacos. **Serves 4**

2 cups meatless crumbles

1 tablespoon coconut oil

1 cup chopped onion

1 bell pepper, seeded and chopped

1½ teaspoons minced garlic

8 ounces mushrooms, sliced

1 head butter lettuce, leaves separated

¼ cup chopped fresh cilantro

½ cup salsa

1 cup shredded cheddar cheese

1 avocado, peeled, pitted, and diced

1. In a medium skillet over medium heat, cook the crumbles until thoroughly warmed. Transfer the crumbles to a medium bowl.

2. In the same skillet, melt the coconut oil and sauté the onion, bell pepper, garlic, and mushrooms for 4 to 5 minutes. Stir the veggie mixture into the crumbles.

3. Divide the mixture equally among the lettuce leaves on four plates.

4. Top the lettuce cups with the cilantro, salsa, cheddar cheese, and avocado.

Tip: If butter lettuce isn't readily available, use romaine or kale instead. They both have hearty leaves that can hold the taco filling.

Per Serving Calories: 316; Total Fat: 19g; Total Carbs: 21g; Fiber: 8g; Net Carbs: 13g; Protein: 22g; Macros: Fat 54%/ Protein 28%/Carbs 18%

Red Pepper–Cauliflower Hummus

Prep time: 10 minutes Cook time: 20 minutes

This easy, keto-friendly hummus is made with roasted cauliflower instead of chickpeas and is perfect for snacking or packing for lunch. Served with cucumber slices, celery sticks, bell pepper strips, cherry tomatoes, keto crackers, or in a lettuce wrap, this dairy-free, low-carb, savory hummus is a crowd-pleaser. **Makes 2½ cups**

1 large head cauliflower, cut into florets

5 tablespoons extra-virgin olive oil or avocado oil, divided

1¾ teaspoons kosher salt, divided

2 tablespoons freshly squeezed lemon juice

6 tablespoons tahini

1 or 2 garlic cloves, peeled

¼ teaspoon freshly ground black pepper

¾ teaspoon ground cumin

¼ cup roasted red pepper

2 to 5 tablespoons water (optional)

1. Preheat the oven to 450°F. Line a baking sheet with parchment paper.

2. In a large bowl, toss the cauliflower with 3 tablespoons olive oil and 1 teaspoon salt. Spread the florets on the baking sheet in a single layer. Roast the cauliflower for about 20 minutes, or until the florets are caramelized and tender. Remove from the oven and cool.

3. In a food processor or high-speed blender, puree the roasted cauliflower, lemon juice, tahini, garlic, remaining ¾ teaspoon salt, black pepper, cumin, roasted red pepper, and remaining 2 tablespoons olive oil until smooth. If the hummus is too thick, add the water, 1 tablespoon at a time, to reach your desired consistency.

Tip: If you prefer a more subtle garlic flavor, you can roast the garlic cloves. Place 2 or 3 unpeeled garlic cloves on a small piece of aluminum foil. Drizzle with a little olive oil, wrap them up, and roast them with the cauliflower. Unwrap the foil, peel the garlic, and add it to the food processor or blender as instructed.

Per Serving (1 tablespoon) Calories: 35; Total Fat: 3g; Total Carbs: 2g; Fiber: 1g; Net Carbs: 1g; Protein: 1g; Macros: Fat 77%/Protein 11%/Carbs 12%

"Everything" Fat Bombs

Prep time: 10 minutes, plus 1 hour 30 minutes to chill

It's true that foods and flavors have trends, and right now it seems as though there is nothing hotter than everything bagel seasoning. This seasoning—a blend of poppy seeds, sesame seeds, dried garlic, dried onion, and salt—is good on just about everything. And if you find yourself craving bread, this recipe will keep you right on track, giving you all the flavors of a savory New York bagel. **Makes 7 fat bombs**

8 ounces cream cheese, at room temperature

2 cups shredded cheddar cheese

1 (2.3-ounce) jar everything bagel seasoning

1. In a medium bowl or food processor, combine the cream cheese and cheddar cheese until well mixed. Put the mixture in the refrigerator to chill for 1 hour.

2. Line a baking sheet with parchment paper. Pour the seasoning onto a plate and set aside.

3. Remove the cheese mixture from the refrigerator and roll it into 1-inch balls. Roll each ball in the seasoning mix until completely covered. Transfer the coated balls to the prepared baking sheet.

4. Place the baking sheet in the refrigerator and chill for 30 minutes.

Tip: Store extra fat bombs in an airtight container (not a plastic bag) so they can retain their shape. They will keep well in the refrigerator for up to 3 days.

Per Serving (1 bomb) Calories: 290; Total Fat: 22g; Total Carbs: 3g; Fiber: 0g; Net Carbs: 3g; Protein: 9g; Macros: Fat 68%/Protein 12%/Carbs 20%

Blue Cheese–Cucumber Bites

Prep time: 10 minutes

If you're a fan of tangy blue cheese, these quick, refreshing cucumber bites are going to be your new obsession. Gorgonzola is a mild blue cheese and can be purchased in the specialty cheese section of many grocery stores. This buttery cheese pairs perfectly with crunchy toasted walnuts and makes for a sinful bite. **Makes 20 bites**

4 ounces cream cheese, at room temperature

3 tablespoons butter, at room temperature

1 cup crumbled Gorgonzola cheese

¼ cup finely chopped toasted walnuts

2 scallions, both white and light green parts, sliced

Pinch kosher salt

1 large English cucumber, sliced in ¼-inch rounds

1. In a small mixing bowl, beat the cream cheese and butter until smooth. Stir in the Gorgonzola, walnuts, scallions, and salt.

2. Spoon the cheese mixture onto the cucumber slices and serve.

Tip: To toast the walnut halves, preheat the oven to 350°F. Place the walnuts in an even layer on a baking sheet lined with parchment paper and toast until fragrant and golden, 8 to 10 minutes. Be sure to stir every few minutes to prevent burning. Remove the nuts from the pan, cool, and chop.

Per Serving (1 bite) Calories: 71; Total Fat: 7g; Total Carbs: 1g; Fiber: <1g; Net Carbs: <1g; Protein: 2g; Macros: Fat 89%/Protein 11%/Carbs 0%

Herbed Mozzarella Sticks

Prep time: 10 minutes Cook time: 20 minutes

Traditional mozzarella sticks are coated with bread crumbs, which adds to their carb count. A simple switch—more cheese!—enables you to still enjoy these treats. Grated almost to a powder, Parmesan is fine enough to coat the mozzarella sticks and crisps up just like bread crumbs. **Serves 8**

½ cup peanut oil

1 cup very finely grated Parmesan cheese

1 tablespoon Italian seasoning

½ teaspoon garlic salt

2 eggs, beaten

8 sticks full-fat string cheese, halved horizontally

1. Pour the peanut oil into a small skillet over high heat. Line a plate with paper towels.

2. While the oil is heating, in a small bowl, mix together the Parmesan cheese, Italian seasoning, and garlic salt. In another small bowl, beat the eggs.

3. Dredge each string cheese stick first in the beaten egg and then in the cheese and herb mixture, rolling the sticks so they are fully coated.

4. Carefully slip 3 or 4 sticks into the hot oil. Cook until all sides are golden brown, about 3 minutes. Transfer to the paper towel–lined plate to drain for a few minutes.

5. Repeat with the remaining cheese sticks. Serve warm.

Per Serving Calories: 280; Total Fat: 25g; Total Carbs: 2g; Fiber: <1g; Net Carbs: 2g; Protein: 12g; Macros: Fat 80%/ Protein 17%/Carbs 3%

Jalapeño Popper Pimento Cheese

Prep time: 15 minutes Cook time: 20 minutes

This spicy, garlicky spread takes just a few minutes to throw together and is super delicious. Served on top of cucumber slices or stuffed in celery, it's the perfect keto snack or quick lunch. You can also use it as a topping on your bun-less burger. **Makes 4 cups**

2 or 3 jalapeño peppers

Avocado oil or bacon fat, for drizzling

4 ounces cream cheese, at room temperature

8 ounces sharp cheddar cheese, shredded

8 ounces Monterey Jack cheese, shredded

½ teaspoon freshly ground black pepper

½ teaspoon granulated garlic

¼ teaspoon paprika

⅓ cup chopped crispy-cooked bacon

1½ tablespoons diced pimentos

½ cup keto-friendly mayonnaise or Three-Minute Mayo (page 178)

1. Preheat the oven to 375°F. Line a small baking sheet with parchment paper.

2. Place the jalapeños on the lined baking sheet and drizzle with the avocado oil. Roast until the jalapeños start to blister and char, 15 to 20 minutes. Remove from the oven and set aside to cool.

3. Once cool, remove the skins and seeds from the jalapeños. Finely chop them and set aside.

4. In a large mixing bowl, combine the cream cheese, cheddar and Monterey Jack cheeses, black pepper, garlic, paprika, bacon, pimentos, mayonnaise, and the desired amount of chopped roasted jalapeño. Mix with a handheld mixer until thoroughly combined.

5. The flavor will improve as the pimento cheese chills and it will firm up as it cools. Add a little more mayo as needed to reach your desired consistency for serving.

Per Serving (¼ cup) Calories: 192; Total Fat: 17g; Total Carbs: 1g; Fiber: <1g; Net Carbs: 1g; Protein: 8g; Macros: Fat 80%/Protein 17%/Carbs 3%

Pickle-Brined Chicken Wings

Prep time: 5 minutes, plus 4 to 6 hours to brine Cook time: 40 minutes

These brined chicken wings get some serious flavor thanks to some ordinary pickle juice and a quick, spicy rub. Feeding a crowd? This recipe can easily be doubled or tripled; just bake the wings in batches to ensure maximum crispiness. **Serves 8**

2 pounds chicken wings

2 cups dill pickle juice

2 teaspoons kosher salt

1 teaspoon freshly ground black pepper

1 teaspoon chili powder

½ teaspoon paprika

1 teaspoon garlic powder

½ teaspoon onion powder

½ teaspoon cayenne pepper (optional)

Ranch Dressing (page 181), for serving

1. Place the chicken wings in a gallon-size zip-top bag and add the pickle juice. Press the air from the bag, seal, and refrigerate for at least 4 to 6 hours.

2. When you're ready to cook, preheat the oven to 425°F. Line a large baking sheet with parchment paper and place a metal baking rack on top.

3. Remove the wings from the bag and pat dry with paper towels. Place in a large bowl. Discard the pickle juice.

4. In a small bowl, combine the salt, black pepper, chili powder, paprika, garlic powder, onion powder, and cayenne pepper (if using) and mix well. Sprinkle the dry wings with the seasoning blend and toss to coat. Place the seasoned wings on the rack.

5. Bake the wings for about 40 minutes, flipping once during cooking. Serve warm with the ranch dressing.

Per Serving Calories: 221; Total Fat: 15g; Total Carbs: 1g; Fiber: <1g; Net Carbs: 1g; Protein: 20g; Macros: Fat 61%/ Protein 36%/Carbs 3%

Loaded Deviled Eggs

Prep time: 10 minutes

Deviled eggs are a keto must! Easy to make and packed with protein and healthy fats, they make a hearty, tasty snack. Hard-boiled eggs—loaded or not—are great to prep ahead and keep on hand for a quick breakfast or snack. **Serves 6**

6 hard-boiled eggs, peeled and halved lengthwise

3 tablespoons keto-friendly mayonnaise or Three-Minute Mayo (page 178)

1½ tablespoons sour cream

3 tablespoons shredded cheddar cheese

2 scallions, both white and green parts, sliced

Pinch kosher salt

⅛ teaspoon freshly ground black pepper

3 bacon slices, cooked crispy and crumbled

1. Remove the yolks from the hard-boiled egg halves and place them in a bowl with the mayonnaise, sour cream, cheddar cheese, scallions, salt, and pepper. Mix until well combined.

2. Spoon the yolk mixture back into the egg whites. Top with the crumbled bacon and serve immediately.

Tip: For perfectly hard-boiled eggs, place the eggs in a single layer in a saucepan. Fill the pot with cool water to about 1 inch above the eggs. Bring the pot to a rolling boil, then cover, remove from the heat, and let the eggs sit in the hot water for 13 minutes. Drain the eggs and cover with cool water and ice until completely cooled. Store unpeeled eggs in the refrigerator until you're ready to use them.

Per Serving Calories: 160; Total Fat: 14g; Total Carbs: 1g; Fiber: <1g; Net Carbs: 1g; Protein: 8g; Macros: Fat 79%/ Protein 20%/Carbs 1%

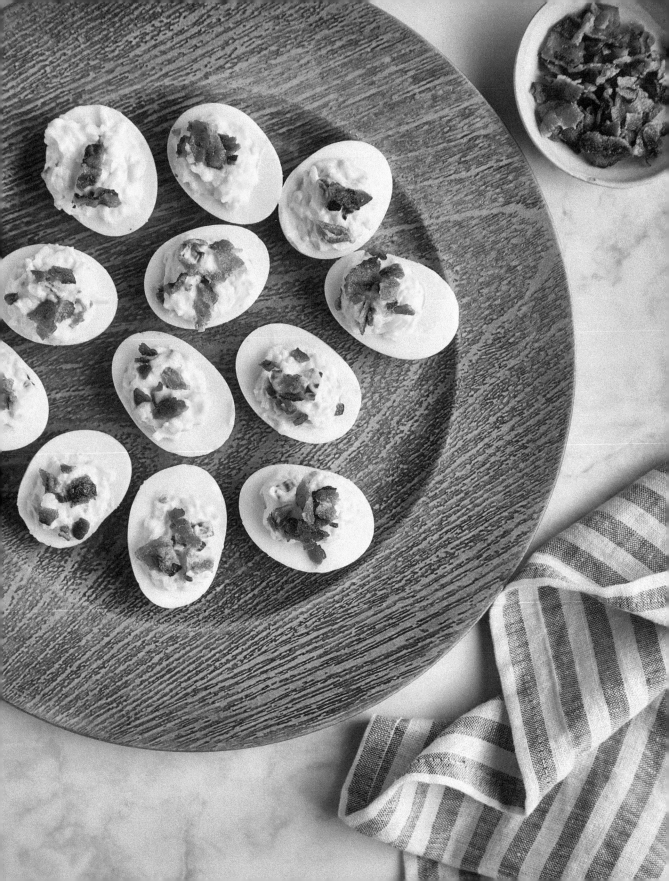

Buffalo Chicken–Stuffed Celery

Prep time: 15 minutes Cook time: 25 minutes

Celery is bland on its own, but with a little buffalo chicken on top, it's a different story. This protein-packed recipe is quick and doesn't require many ingredients. It works well to prepare in advance and bring to work for a delicious snack. For the buffalo hot sauce, I like Frank's RedHot; pick what you like, but beware of added sugar. **Makes 20 pieces**

1 teaspoon extra-virgin olive oil, plus more for greasing

2 (6-ounce) boneless, skinless chicken breasts

1 teaspoon kosher salt, plus more for seasoning

½ teaspoon freshly ground black pepper, plus more for seasoning

½ cup shredded cheddar cheese

¼ cup keto-friendly mayonnaise or Three-Minute Mayo (page 178)

3 tablespoons buffalo hot sauce

½ teaspoon garlic powder

10 celery stalks, cut into 3-inch pieces

1. Preheat the oven to 400°F. Lightly grease a baking sheet with olive oil.

2. Toss the chicken breasts with the olive oil and season with salt and pepper.

3. Place the chicken on the baking sheet and bake for 22 to 25 minutes, or until the internal temperature reaches 165°F. Let rest for 5 minutes, then shred the meat using two forks.

4. In a large bowl, mix together the shredded chicken, cheddar cheese, mayonnaise, buffalo sauce, salt, pepper, and the garlic powder until combined.

5. Fill each celery stalk with the chicken mixture.

Tip: If you don't have celery, bell peppers work in a pinch and have a satisfying crunch.

Per Serving (2 pieces) Calories: 110; Total Fat: 8g; Total Carbs: 2g; Fiber: 1g; Net Carbs: 1g; Protein: 9g; Macros: Fat 65%/Protein 33%/Carbs 2%

"Corn Dog" Bites

Prep time: 10 minutes Cook time: 20 minutes

Get your fast food fix with these fun keto "corn dog" bites. They're great for packing in lunches or for snacking. Serve them with mustard or sugar-free ketchup. Just read the label on your hot dogs to check the carb count and make sure there's no added sugar. **Makes 32 bites**

5 tablespoons butter, melted, plus more for greasing

4 hot dogs

1 cup almond flour

2½ tablespoons coconut flour

½ teaspoon kosher salt

2½ teaspoons baking powder

¼ teaspoon baking soda

¼ teaspoon garlic powder

¼ teaspoon onion powder

1½ teaspoons granulated 1:1 sweetener

4 eggs

2 tablespoons sour cream

⅔ cup shredded sharp cheddar cheese

1. Preheat the oven to 375°F. Grease two metal or silicone 24-cup mini muffin pans with butter.

2. Cut each hot dog into 8 pieces and set aside.

3. In a medium bowl, combine the almond flour, coconut flour, salt, baking powder, baking soda, garlic powder, onion powder, and sweetener and stir to combine. Add the eggs, sour cream, and butter and whisk until thoroughly incorporated. Fold in the cheddar cheese.

4. Place about 1 tablespoon of batter in each muffin cup, then press a piece of hot dog into the center of each cup. Bake for 18 to 20 minutes, or until golden. Cool in the pan for 10 minutes, then remove to cool on a rack.

Tip: If you don't have two mini muffin pans, prepare these bites in two batches.

Per Serving (1 bite) Calories: 75; Total Fat: 7g; Total Carbs: 2g; Fiber: 1g; Net Carbs: 1g; Protein: 3g; Macros: Fat 84%/ Protein 16%/Carbs 0%

Pepperoni Pizza Rolls

Prep time: 12 minutes Cook time: 20 minutes

Soft, cheesy, and loaded with pizza flavor, these easy pepperoni pizza rolls are always a winner, especially with kids, and they take just a few minutes to put together. They're perfect for entertaining and ideal for packing in lunches or having in the refrigerator to fend off cravings. Use jarred marinara to keep this recipe under 30 minutes, or whip up a batch of Quick Marinara Sauce (page 183) for extra homemade flavor. **Makes 12 pizza rolls**

2 tablespoons butter, melted, plus more for greasing

1 batch Keto Dough (page 186)

4 tablespoons sugar-free marinara or Quick Marinara Sauce (page 183), divided, plus more for dipping

2 cups shredded mozzarella cheese, divided

4 ounces thinly sliced pepperoni, divided

2 tablespoons grated Parmesan cheese, divided

1 garlic clove, minced

1. Preheat the oven to 375°F. Lightly grease a standard 12-cup muffin pan with butter.

2. Divide the dough in half and work with one piece at a time. Roll the dough between two pieces of parchment paper to form a rectangle about ¼ inch thick. Remove the top piece of parchment.

3. Spread 2 tablespoons marinara sauce on top of the dough. Evenly sprinkle 1 cup mozzarella cheese over the marinara sauce. Layer half of the sliced pepperoni on top of the cheese, then sprinkle with 1 tablespoon Parmesan cheese. Starting with the long end, roll up the dough, jelly roll–style, using the parchment paper for assistance if needed, and pinch to seal the edge.

4. Using a serrated knife, cut the roll into 6 pieces and place, cut-side down, in the prepared muffin cups. Repeat steps 2 through 4 with the remaining portion of dough.

5. Combine the butter and garlic and brush over the top of each pizza roll. Bake for 15 to 18 minutes, or until golden. Let cool for 10 minutes in the pan, then remove. Serve warm with more marinara sauce for dipping.

Tip: The possibilities for these pizza rolls are endless! Not a pepperoni fan? Swap it for diced ham or Canadian bacon, browned Italian sausage, or even leftover browned ground beef.

Per Serving (1 roll) Calories: 268; Total Fat: 22g; Total Carbs: 5g; Fiber: 2g; Net Carbs: 3g; Protein: 13g; Macros: Fat 74%/Protein 19%/Carbs 7%

Cheesy Sausage Balls

Prep time: 7 minutes Cook time: 20 minutes

Sausage balls were an appetizer staple when I was growing up, and this keto version is even better than the original. Quick and easy to prepare, they make a hearty keto snack, appetizer, or even a fast lunch. Make a double batch and freeze them for up to one month. **Makes 24 sausage balls**

1 pound hot breakfast sausage

1 egg

¾ cup almond flour

1 cup shredded cheddar cheese

¼ cup grated Parmesan cheese

2 teaspoons baking powder

¼ teaspoon kosher salt

½ teaspoon garlic powder

2 scallions, both white and green parts, sliced

1. Preheat the oven to 375°F. Line a baking sheet with parchment paper.

2. In a medium bowl, mix together the sausage, egg, almond flour, cheddar and Parmesan cheeses, baking powder, salt, garlic powder, and scallions. Work everything with a spoon or your hands until the ingredients are thoroughly combined.

3. Using a cookie scoop or spoon, shape the mixture into walnut-size balls (about 1½ tablespoons each) and place them on the lined baking sheet. Bake for 20 to 22 minutes, or until golden brown.

Per Serving (3 sausage balls) Calories: 329; Total Fat: 30g; Total Carbs: 2g; Fiber: <1g; Net Carbs: 2g; Protein: 14g; Macros: Fat 82%/Protein 17%/Carbs 1%

Cajun Roast Beef Dip

Prep time: 10 minutes, plus 1 hour to chill

This savory roast beef dip was always on the appetizer table when I was growing up, and for good reason: It's delicious and so easy to make. These days, there are a number of quality roast beef options at the deli counter in your grocery store that will work perfectly in this dip. Just avoid any with added sugar, MSG, or other additives. Serve this dip with veggies or Cheesy Crackers (page 185). **Makes 2½ cups**

8 ounces thinly sliced roast beef deli meat, chopped

¼ cup finely diced red onion

2 cups sour cream

½ teaspoon Cajun seasoning

1. In a medium bowl, combine the roast beef, onion, sour cream, and Cajun seasoning. Stir well to combine.

2. Cover and chill for at least 1 hour before serving.

Per Serving (1 tablespoon) Calories: 30; Total Fat: 2g; Total Carbs: 1g; Fiber: 0g; Net Carbs: 1g; Protein: 1g; Macros: Fat 60%/Protein 13%/Carbs 27%

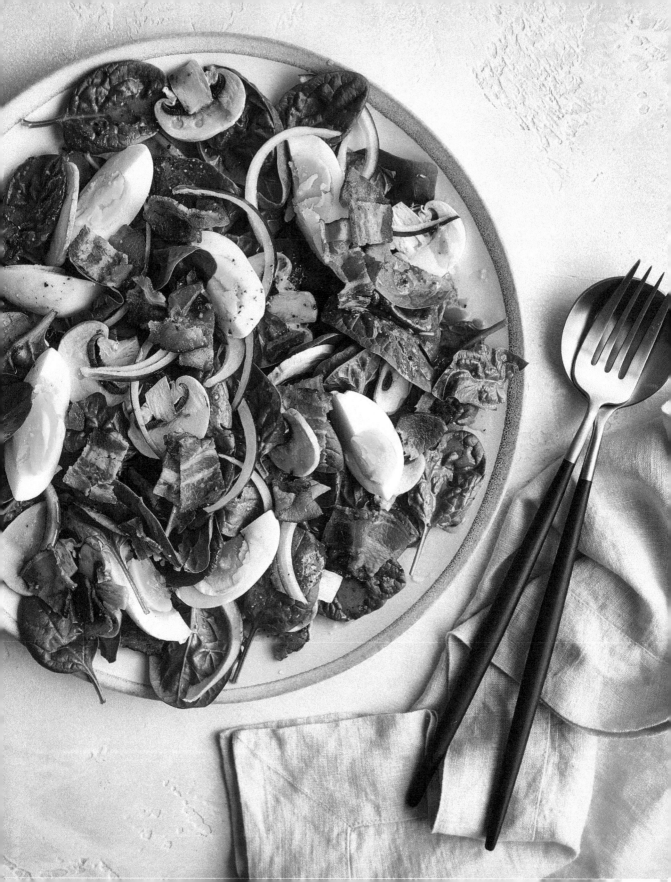

CHAPTER 4

Salads and Soups

Spinach Salad with Warm Bacon Dressing, page 65

5 INGREDIENTS OR FEWER, NO-COOK, VEGETARIAN

Tomato and Brie Salad

Prep time: 15 minutes, plus 30 minutes to marinate

This simple salad is perfect for summer when tomatoes, zucchini, and basil are in season, and it pairs perfectly with grilled steak or chicken as a quick and easy side. Plus, it's best served at room temperature so it's perfect for an outdoor cookout, barbecue, or potluck. Brie is a soft cheese with an edible white rind that you can remove, if desired. **Serves 4**

1 (8-ounce) round
brie cheese

2 large tomatoes, cut into
½-inch pieces

1 medium zucchini, cut into
½-inch pieces

⅓ cup chopped fresh basil

3 garlic cloves,
finely chopped

¼ cup extra-virgin olive oil or
avocado oil

¼ teaspoon kosher salt

½ teaspoon freshly ground
black pepper

1. Remove the rind from the brie using a sharp knife, if desired.

2. In a medium bowl, toss together the brie, tomatoes, zucchini, basil, garlic, olive oil, salt, and pepper.

3. Cover and let stand at room temperature for at least 30 minutes before serving.

Tip: The rind on brie is completely edible and delicious, but some people just don't like it. The secret to removing it is to dip a knife in hot water for a few seconds, dry with a towel, and cut, repeating as needed.

Per Serving Calories: 338; Total Fat: 30g; Total Carbs: 6g; Fiber: 2g; Net Carbs: 4g; Protein: 13g; Macros: Fat 80%/Protein 15%/Carbs 5%

Marinated Vegetable Salad

Prep time: 15 minutes

This bright and tangy salad is one of my favorite summer sides. It's a tasty combination of avocado, tomatoes, cucumbers, artichoke hearts, and hearts of palm, all marinated in a quick, lemony garlic dressing. **Serves 6**

½ cup extra-virgin olive oil

2 or 3 garlic cloves,
finely minced

2 tablespoons white
wine vinegar

3 tablespoons freshly
squeezed lemon
juice, divided

½ teaspoon granulated
1:1 sweetener

½ teaspoon mustard powder

¼ teaspoon Italian seasoning

½ teaspoon kosher salt

⅛ teaspoon freshly ground
black pepper

2 large ripe avocados, peeled,
pitted, and diced

1 (14-ounce) can hearts of
palm, drained and sliced

1 (14-ounce) can artichoke
hearts, drained and
quartered

1½ cups halved grape
tomatoes

2 English
cucumbers, quartered
and diced

1. In a jar, combine the olive oil, garlic, vinegar, 2 tablespoons lemon juice, the sweetener, mustard powder, Italian seasoning, salt, and pepper. Cover tightly with a lid and shake. Set aside.

2. In a medium bowl, sprinkle the avocado with the remaining 1 tablespoon lemon juice and toss gently to coat. Add the hearts of palm, artichoke hearts, tomatoes, and cucumbers. Pour the dressing over the vegetables and toss the salad gently to combine.

Tip: This salad is great served the next day as leftovers; the flavors just get better as it sits. That being said, the cool refrigerator may cause the olive oil to solidify overnight. Simply remove the salad from the fridge and let it come to room temperature before serving.

Per Serving Calories: 325; Total Fat: 28g; Total Carbs: 18g; Fiber: 8g; Net Carbs: 10g; Protein: 5g; Macros: Fat 77%/ Protein 6%/Carbs 17%

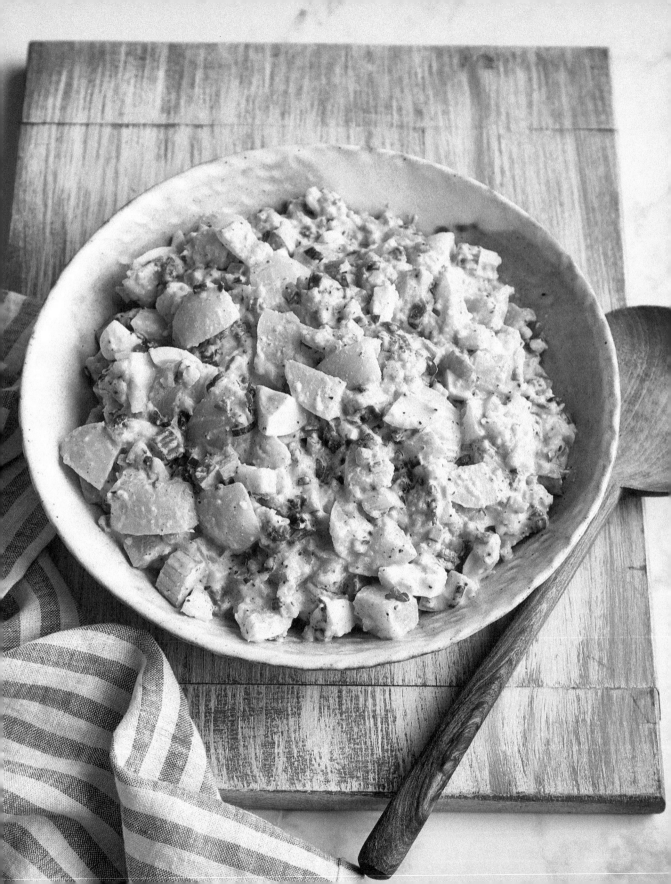

Classic Fauxtato Salad

Prep time: 20 minutes Cook time: 10 minutes

This Southern-style keto "potato" salad has all the comforting flavors of the old-school potato salad you grew up enjoying, but with a fraction of the carbs. Using turnips as the base creates a delicious low-carb side that will fool even potato lovers. Prepare in advance for maximum flavor. **Serves 8**

2 pounds turnips, peeled and cut into ½-inch pieces

Kosher salt

⅔ cup keto-friendly mayonnaise or Three-Minute Mayo (page 178)

3 tablespoons yellow mustard

¼ teaspoon onion powder

⅛ teaspoon granulated garlic

¼ teaspoon paprika

¼ teaspoon celery salt

¼ teaspoon freshly ground black pepper

4 scallions, both white and green parts, sliced

3 hard-boiled eggs, peeled and chopped

½ cup diced celery

⅓ cup chopped no-sugar-added pickles

3 tablespoons diced pimentos

1. Line a large baking sheet with a clean dish towel or paper towels.

2. Place the turnips in a medium pot and cover with water. Lightly salt the water and bring the turnips to a boil over high heat. Cook for about 10 minutes, or until fork-tender. Drain the turnips and spread them out on the baking sheet. Put the turnips in the refrigerator to cool for about 10 minutes, or until they reach room temperature.

3. Meanwhile, in a small bowl, combine the mayonnaise, mustard, onion powder, garlic, paprika, celery salt, and pepper. Mix well and set aside.

4. Once the turnips are cooled, use a potato masher to smash them right on the baking sheet to the desired chunkiness. Replace the paper towel under the turnips, if needed. Continue to remove the excess water by pressing the turnips gently between paper towels or dish towels.

continued >

5. Place the mashed turnips in a large bowl and add the scallions, eggs, celery, pickles, and pimentos. Toss well to combine. Add the mayonnaise dressing and gently mix until well combined. Cover and refrigerate until serving time.

Per Serving Calories: 198; Total Fat: 17g; Total Carbs: 9g; Fiber: 3g; Net Carbs: 6g; Protein: 4g; Macros: Fat 77%/Protein 8%/Carbs 15%

Jalapeño Coleslaw

Prep time: 15 minutes

A delicious keto coleslaw is a great thing to have in your recipe arsenal, especially during the grilling and barbecue season. This tangy, slightly sweet, spiced-up slaw is amazing paired with anything grilled or smoked. It complements a ton of dishes from barbecued brisket and chicken to blackened fish and grilled seafood. **Serves 4**

1 (1-pound) bag coleslaw mix or 1 pound green cabbage, finely shredded

¼ cup thinly sliced red onion

2½ tablespoons finely diced jalapeño pepper

3 scallions, both white and green parts, sliced

¼ cup sour cream

¼ cup keto-friendly mayonnaise or Three-Minute Mayo (page 178)

2¼ teaspoons apple cider vinegar

1½ teaspoons yellow mustard

1 tablespoon granulated 1:1 sweetener

¼ teaspoon ground cumin

¼ teaspoon granulated garlic

¼ teaspoon paprika

¼ teaspoon kosher salt

1. In a large bowl, toss together the coleslaw mix, onion, jalapeño, and scallions.

2. In a small bowl, combine the sour cream, mayonnaise, vinegar, mustard, sweetener, cumin, garlic, paprika, and salt. Stir well.

3. Pour the dressing over the slaw and gently toss to coat. Cover and refrigerate until serving time.

Per Serving Calories: 169; Total Fat: 14g; Total Carbs: 13g; Fiber: 3g; Net Carbs: 4g; Protein: 3g; Macros: Fat 74%/ Protein 7%/Carbs 19%

Asian-Inspired Chopped Salad

Prep time: 15 minutes

This easy Asian-inspired chopped salad is tossed in a quick, flavor-packed sesame dressing. Serve it as a side dish or as a main course topped with the protein of your choice. **Serves 6**

1½ teaspoons minced fresh ginger

2 garlic cloves, grated

2 tablespoons tamari, soy sauce, or coconut aminos

3 tablespoons apple cider vinegar

1½ teaspoons sesame oil

⅓ cup avocado oil

1 tablespoon freshly squeezed lime juice

1½ teaspoons granulated 1:1 sweetener

2 cups chopped romaine lettuce

4 cups thinly sliced Napa cabbage

½ red bell pepper, seeded and thinly cut into 1-inch strips

3 scallions, both white and green parts, sliced

1 cup English cucumber, cut into half-moons

3 tablespoons chopped fresh cilantro

3 tablespoons chopped roasted salted peanuts

1. In a small bowl, combine the ginger, garlic, tamari, vinegar, sesame oil, avocado oil, lime juice, and sweetener and whisk well to combine. Set aside.

2. In a large bowl, toss together the lettuce, cabbage, bell pepper, scallions, cucumber, and cilantro.

3. Pour the dressing over the salad and toss to coat. Sprinkle with the chopped peanuts and serve immediately.

Tip: Make this an Asian-Inspired Chopped Chicken Salad by adding 3 cups of chopped cooked chicken to the vegetables before tossing with the dressing. Shrimp or salmon would also work well.

Per Serving Calories: 169; Total Fat: 16g; Total Carbs: 6g; Fiber: 2g; Net Carbs: 4g; Protein: 3g; Macros: Fat 85%/Protein 7%/Carbs 8%

Spinach Salad with Warm Bacon Dressing

Prep time: 10 minutes Cook time: 10 minutes

A warm dressing on cool greens may sound like an unusual combination, but this might become one of your favorite salads ever. To make the dressing lightly sweet, I use a small amount of zero-carb sweetener. The warm bacon fat helps it dissolve, and it's the perfect complement to the tangy red wine vinegar. **Serves 6**

12 bacon slices

5 tablespoons red wine vinegar

1 teaspoon granulated 1:1 sweetener

1 teaspoon Dijon mustard

¼ teaspoon kosher salt

¼ teaspoon freshly ground black pepper

12 ounces baby spinach

4 hard-boiled eggs, peeled and sliced

6 large button mushrooms, thinly sliced

1 small red onion, very thinly sliced

1. Cook the bacon, chop, and set aside.

2. Transfer ¼ cup of bacon fat to a small saucepan over low heat. Add the vinegar, sweetener, mustard, salt, and pepper. Whisk vigorously until the sweetener is dissolved and the fat and vinegar blend to form a vinaigrette. Let sit over very low heat to keep warm.

3. In a large salad bowl, gently toss together the spinach, eggs, mushrooms, onion, and bacon.

4. When you're ready to serve, drizzle the warm vinaigrette over the salad and toss again. Serve immediately.

Tip: If you'll be making this salad ahead of time, toss the ingredients and store in a covered container in the refrigerator. Put the dressing in a bowl, cover with plastic wrap, and store in the refrigerator. Warm up the dressing in the microwave just before serving.

Per Serving Calories: 146; Total Fat: 9g; Total Carbs: 5g; Fiber: 2g; Net Carbs: 3g; Protein: 12g; Macros: Fat 55%/ Protein 33%/Carbs 12%

Black and Blue Salad

Prep time: 10 minutes Cook time: 5 minutes

The combination of spicy blackened steak, tangy Gorgonzola cheese, creamy avocado, and crunchy pecans creates an explosion of flavor and textures that will blow your mind. Flank steak has an amazing flavor and a super quick cook time, but feel free to use any cut of steak or even leftover steak you have on hand to top this flavorful salad. **Serves 4**

1 pound flank steak, at room temperature

Blackening or Cajun seasoning, for seasoning

1 tablespoon bacon fat or avocado oil

4 cups mixed lettuce greens

4 ounces crumbled Gorgonzola cheese

1 cup halved grape tomatoes

¼ red onion, sliced

1 avocado, peeled, pitted, and diced

¼ cup toasted pecan pieces

Your favorite salad dressing, for topping

1. Season the flank steak generously with the blackening or Cajun seasoning.

2. In a heavy-bottomed skillet, heat the bacon fat over medium-high heat. When the pan is hot, sear the steak for 2 to 3 minutes per side, or until it's cooked the way you like. Remove from the heat, cover with aluminum foil, and let rest while you assemble the rest of the salad.

3. In a large bowl, toss together the greens, Gorgonzola, tomatoes, onion, and avocado. Thinly slice the steak against the grain and place on top of the salad. Sprinkle with toasted pecans and serve topped with your favorite salad dressing.

Tip: Blackening is done in a very hot pan, and that produces a lot of smoke. Be sure to have your overhead exhaust fan on while you're cooking the steak.

Per Serving Calories: 454; Total Fat: 32g; Total Carbs: 10g; Fiber: 5g; Net Carbs: 5g; Protein: 33g; Macros: Fat 63%/ Protein 29%/Carbs 8%

Broccoli and Cheddar Soup

Prep time: 10 minutes Cook time: 25 minutes

Not everyone loves broccoli, but hopefully we can agree on one thing: Broccoli tastes a heck of a lot better with some cheddar cheese on it! This is a simple one-pot recipe that's perfect to eat with a big, juicy steak. You can use fresh broccoli if you have it in your refrigerator. **Serves 6**

2 tablespoons extra-virgin olive oil

1 (14-ounce) package frozen broccoli florets

½ onion, diced

2 garlic cloves, minced

1 teaspoon kosher salt

½ teaspoon freshly ground black pepper

4 cups chicken stock

1 cup heavy (whipping) cream

¼ cup cream cheese, at room temperature

2 cups shredded cheddar cheese

1. In a large stockpot, heat the olive oil over medium heat. Add the broccoli, onion, garlic, salt, and pepper. Sauté until the broccoli is soft and the onion and garlic are translucent and tender, 10 to 15 minutes.

2. Add the chicken stock and heavy cream to the pot. Stir, then bring to a simmer. Reduce the heat to low and add the cream cheese.

3. Add the cheddar cheese, 1 cup at a time, stirring after each cup until the cheese is melted and the soup is smooth. Remove from the heat and serve.

Tip: If cheddar's not your jam, try Gouda or mozzarella cheese.

Per Serving Calories: 374; Total Fat: 33g; Total Carbs: 7g; Fiber: 2g; Net Carbs: 5g; Protein: 14g; Macros: Fat 79%/ Protein 15%/Carbs 6%

Coconut Veggie Curry Soup

Prep time: 15 minutes Cook time: 30 minutes

This aromatic curry has a great flavor and will likely make it into your weekly rotation of favorites. Curries are often served with rice or naan, but for keto we can just bulk up the vegetables a little and enjoy this thick soup. **Serves 4**

2 tablespoons extra-virgin olive oil

½ yellow onion, diced

3 garlic cloves, minced

1½ teaspoons minced fresh ginger

1 teaspoon garam masala

1 teaspoon curry powder

1 teaspoon ground cumin

1 (14-ounce) can no-sugar-added diced tomatoes

3 (14-ounce) cans full-fat coconut milk

1 cauliflower head, cut into florets

2 large zucchini, diced

¼ cup chopped cashews

1. In a stockpot, warm the olive oil over medium-high heat. Add the onion and sauté for 2 to 3 minutes. Stir in the garlic, ginger, garam masala, curry powder, cumin, and tomatoes with their juices. Cook for 2 minutes.

2. Pour in the coconut milk and bring the mixture to a low simmer. Reduce the heat to low and simmer for 5 minutes. Stir in the cauliflower and zucchini and simmer for an additional 20 minutes.

3. Top with the chopped cashews and serve.

Tip: Feel free to switch up the veggies as desired, but make sure to stay away from starchy ingredients, such as corn and potatoes.

Per Serving Calories: 764; Total Fat: 68g; Total Carbs: 38g; Fiber: 10g; Net Carbs: 28g; Protein: 13g; Macros: Fat 80%/Protein 7%/Carbs 13%

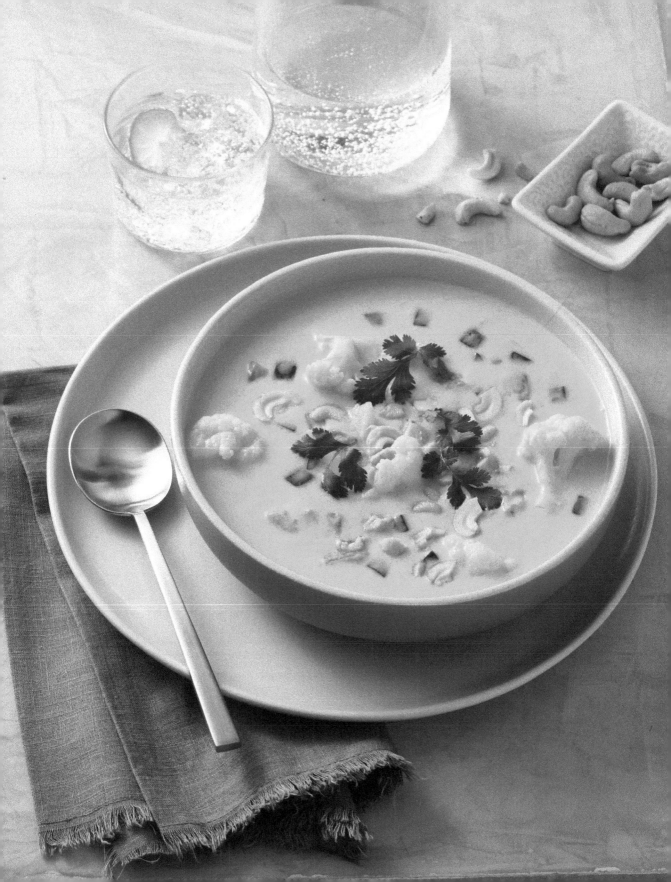

Creamy Zucchini-Poblano Soup

Prep time: 10 minutes Cook time: 25 minutes

I love the combination of zucchini, poblano peppers, and smoky cumin in this simple, velvety soup. Poblanos are a mild chile pepper with a sweet, fruity flavor when cooked. You can easily find them at most grocery stores. This simple soup pairs perfectly with chicken and seafood dishes and is ideal to serve as an appetizer or as a light lunch or dinner with a green salad. **Serves 6**

3 tablespoons butter

½ cup diced onion

2 garlic cloves, sliced

3 medium zucchini, diced

1 poblano pepper, seeded and diced

½ teaspoon ground cumin

1 cup chicken or vegetable stock or bone broth

1 cup water

1 teaspoon kosher salt

½ teaspoon freshly ground black pepper

½ cup heavy (whipping) cream

Optional garnishes: chopped fresh cilantro, lime wedges, and sour cream

1. In a Dutch oven or stockpot, melt the butter over medium heat and add the onion, garlic, zucchini, poblano pepper, and cumin. Sauté for about 10 minutes, or until the onion is translucent.

2. Add the stock, water, salt, and black pepper. Bring the mixture to a boil and simmer for another 10 minutes.

3. Using an immersion blender, puree the soup in the pot. Or carefully transfer the mixture to a countertop blender and blend until smooth. (When blending hot liquids, remove the cap from the blender lid and cover the hole with a towel.) Then return the soup to the pot. Stir in the heavy cream. Taste and adjust the seasoning as needed.

4. If desired, top with chopped cilantro, a lime wedge, and a dollop of sour cream and serve.

Per Serving Calories: 147; Total Fat: 13g; Total Carbs: 6g; Fiber: 1g; Net Carbs: 5g; Protein: 3g; Macros: Fat 79%/ Protein 8%/Carbs 13%

Tomato-Basil Soup

Prep time: 5 minutes Cook time: 25 minutes

Bursting with rich tomato flavor, this creamy and flavorful soup is a family favorite and a million times better than any store-bought version. On the table in about 30 minutes, tomato-basil soup requires no fussy preparation. Be sure to use good-quality canned tomatoes to avoid any metallic after-taste that can sometimes accompany canned tomatoes. Serve this soup topped with fresh basil and extra Parmesan cheese with Garlic-Cheddar Biscuits (page 99) on the side. **Serves 5**

2 tablespoons butter

¼ cup diced onions

2 garlic cloves, roughly chopped

1 (28-ounce) can whole tomatoes

2 cups chicken stock or bone broth

1 tablespoon granulated 1:1 sweetener

2½ teaspoons dried basil

½ teaspoon dried oregano

½ teaspoon kosher salt

¼ teaspoon freshly ground black pepper

½ cup grated Parmesan cheese

½ cup heavy (whipping) cream

1. Melt the butter in a Dutch oven or stockpot over medium heat. Add the onions and sauté until they are translucent but not brown, about 5 minutes. Add the garlic and cook for another minute.

2. Add the tomatoes with their juices, chicken stock, sweetener, basil, oregano, salt, and pepper. Using a spoon, break up the chunks of tomato, then simmer over low heat for 12 to 15 minutes.

3. Using an immersion blender, puree the soup in the pot. Or carefully transfer the tomato mixture to a countertop blender and blend until smooth. (When blending hot liquids, remove the cap from the blender lid and cover the hole with a towel.) Return the soup to the pot. Stir in the Parmesan cheese and heavy cream. Taste and adjust the seasoning as needed.

Per Serving Calories: 211; Total Fat: 16g; Total Carbs: 13g; Fiber: 2g; Net Carbs: 11g; Protein: 5g; Macros: Fat 68%/Protein 14%/Carbs 18%

Beef and Vegetable Soup

Prep time: 10 minutes Cook time: 1 hour 15 minutes

A hearty pot of soup is one of my favorite things to cook and also happens to be the perfect one-pot meal. Comforting and satisfying, a steaming bowl of soup has the power to restore. This soup, full of veggies and tender beef, is comfort food at its finest. And the leftovers are even better. **Serves 6**

3 tablespoons bacon fat or avocado oil

1½ pounds beef stew meat or cubed chuck roast

1½ teaspoons kosher salt, divided

½ teaspoon freshly ground black pepper

1 teaspoon granulated garlic

½ cup diced onion

1 cup diced celery

6 cups beef stock or bone broth

1 (14 ounce-can) diced tomatoes

1 teaspoon dried basil

1 teaspoon dried oregano

2 teaspoon dried parsley

8 ounces turnips, peeled and cut into ½-inch pieces

1 cup frozen green beans

2 cups chopped green cabbage

1. In a large stockpot or Dutch oven, heat the bacon fat over medium-high heat. Season the beef with 1 teaspoon salt, the pepper, and garlic and add half the meat to the pot. Cook the beef for 4 to 5 minutes, until browned on all sides. Remove from the pot and cook the remaining beef in the same way. Remove the beef from the pot and set aside.

2. Put the onion and celery in the pot and sauté for 4 to 5 minutes. Deglaze the pot with the stock, scraping up any browned bit from the bottom, and add the tomatoes with their juices, basil, oregano, parsley, and remaining ½ teaspoon salt. Then add the browned beef to the pot.

3. Bring the soup to a boil, cover, and reduce the heat to low. Simmer for 35 to 40 minutes.

4. Add the turnips, green beans, and cabbage to the pot. Bring to a boil, reduce the heat, cover, and continue to simmer for another 20 minutes. Taste and adjust the seasoning as needed.

Tip: To shorten the cook time, use browned ground beef and reduce the simmer time in step 3 to 20 minutes.

Per Serving Calories: 340; Total Fat: 20g; Total Carbs: 12g; Fiber: 4g; Net Carbs: 8g; Protein: 27g; Macros: Fat 53%/ Protein 32%/Carbs 15%

Homestyle Chicken and "Rice" Soup

Prep time: 10 minutes Cook time: 30 minutes

Rich and flavorful, this chicken soup is perfect for dinner on a cool evening or to have on hand when you're feeling under the weather. All types of rice are off-limits on keto, so I used cauliflower rice to keep this comforting soup keto-friendly. Use bone broth or a high-quality stock. **Serves 6**

2 tablespoons avocado oil or bacon fat

½ cup diced onions

1 cup diced celery, with the leaves

1½ teaspoons kosher salt, divided

4 boneless, skinless chicken thighs, cut into ½-inch pieces

½ teaspoon freshly ground black pepper

1½ teaspoons granulated garlic

6 cups chicken bone broth

½ teaspoon dried thyme

½ teaspoon poultry seasoning

1 tablespoon dried parsley

1 bay leaf

⅓ cup sliced scallions, both white and green parts

2 (12-ounce) packages frozen cauliflower rice

1. In a large stockpot or Dutch oven, heat the avocado oil over medium-high heat. Add the onions, celery, and ½ teaspoon salt and sauté for 2 to 3 minutes.

2. Add the chicken, remaining 1 teaspoon salt, the pepper, and garlic and cook for 4 to 5 minutes, or until the chicken is golden.

3. Deglaze the pan with the chicken broth, scraping up any browned bits from the bottom.

4. Reduce the heat to a simmer and add the thyme, poultry seasoning, parsley, and bay leaf. Simmer for 10 to 15 minutes, or until the chicken is done. Stir in the scallions and cauliflower rice and simmer for another 5 minutes. Remove the bay leaf before serving.

Per Serving Calories: 219; Total Fat: 10g; Total Carbs: 9g; Fiber: 4g; Net Carbs: 5g; Protein: 25g; Macros: Fat 37%/Protein 46%/Carbs 17%

Spicy Thai-Inspired Shrimp Soup

Prep time: 5 minutes Cook time: 25 minutes

There are no Thai restaurants within hours of us, so our only option is to make this favorite at home. Lucky for us, it couldn't be easier. This Thai-inspired soup is all about the broth; the combination of red curry, garlic, ginger, lime, coconut, and shrimp creates an explosion of flavor. To keep things quick and easy, use frozen shrimp that are already peeled and deveined. **Serves 6**

1 tablespoon coconut oil

½ cup diced onion

½ cup diced red bell pepper

½ teaspoon kosher salt

1 teaspoon minced garlic

1 tablespoon grated fresh ginger

3½ tablespoons no-added-sugar red curry paste

3½ cups chicken, seafood, or vegetable stock

1 (13-ounce) can full-fat coconut milk

2 teaspoons granulated 1:1 sweetener

¼ teaspoon grated lime zest

1 pound raw medium or small shrimp, peeled, deveined, and tails removed

1 tablespoon freshly squeezed lime juice (about 1 lime)

3 tablespoons chopped fresh cilantro

1. In a stockpot or Dutch oven, melt the coconut oil over medium-high heat. Add the onion and bell pepper and cook for 4 to 5 minutes, or until the onions are translucent. Add the salt, garlic, ginger, and red curry paste and cook for another minute, stirring constantly.

2. Reduce the heat to medium, stir in the stock, and simmer for about 10 minutes. Add the coconut milk, sweetener, and lime zest. Simmer for another 5 minutes.

3. Add the shrimp to the broth and cook for 2 to 3 minutes, or until the shrimp are pink and cooked through. Taste and adjust the salt as needed.

4. Stir in the lime juice and cilantro and remove from the heat.

Tip: This soup is incredible as-is, but if you want a bit more texture, serve it with your favorite rice alternative stirred in.

Per Serving Calories: 196; Total Fat: 13g; Total Carbs: 11g; Fiber: 2g; Net Carbs: 9g; Protein: 12g; Macros: Fat 60%/ Protein 24%/Carbs 16%

Zuppa Toscana (Sausage and Kale Soup)

Prep time: 10 minutes Cook time: 45 minutes

The name of this classic comfort soup means "Tuscan soup." The star is always kale, but traditional versions include potatoes, beans, and sometimes bread or pasta. This keto version uses cauliflower instead. Kale adds a nutritional boost, but you can easily swap it for baby spinach. Parmesan cheese is the perfect garnish. **Serves 6**

8 ounces bacon, cut into 1-inch pieces

1 pound hot Italian sausage, casings removed

1 medium onion, diced

3 garlic cloves, minced

5 cups chicken stock

1 head cauliflower, stemmed and chopped

3 cups stemmed and chopped kale or baby spinach

½ cup heavy (whipping) cream

½ cup grated Parmesan cheese

1. In a large soup pot, brown the bacon over medium-high heat for 5 to 7 minutes, or until crispy. Using a slotted spoon or fork, transfer the bacon to a paper towel–lined plate. Pour off all but 2 tablespoons of the fat. Reduce the heat to medium.

2. Add the sausage to the pot and cook until browned, about 5 minutes, breaking up the sausage with a wooden spoon. Add the onion and garlic and sauté until the onions are translucent, about 7 minutes. Stir frequently to prevent the garlic from burning.

3. Add the stock. Use the wooden spoon to scrape and deglaze the bottom of the pot. Cover and simmer for 10 minutes.

4. Add the cauliflower. Cover and simmer for 10 minutes, or until the cauliflower is soft.

continued >

5. Add the kale, heavy cream, and bacon and simmer for 5 minutes, or until the kale wilts. Serve in large bowls, garnished with the Parmesan cheese.

Tip: To make this soup in a multicooker, follow the recipe as written but use the Sauté setting for the bacon, sausage, and vegetable steps. Add about 1 cup of broth and use a wooden spoon to scrape the bottom and deglaze the pot. Add the remaining broth and the other ingredients (except the cream and kale). Secure the lid and cook on low pressure for 15 minutes, using a quick release at the end of the cook time. Afterward, use the Sauté setting for 5 minutes while stirring in the cream and kale.

Per Serving Calories: 559; Total Fat: 44g; Total Carbs: 12g; Fiber: 3g; Net Carbs: 9g; Protein: 30g; Macros: Fat 71%/ Protein 21%/Carbs 8%

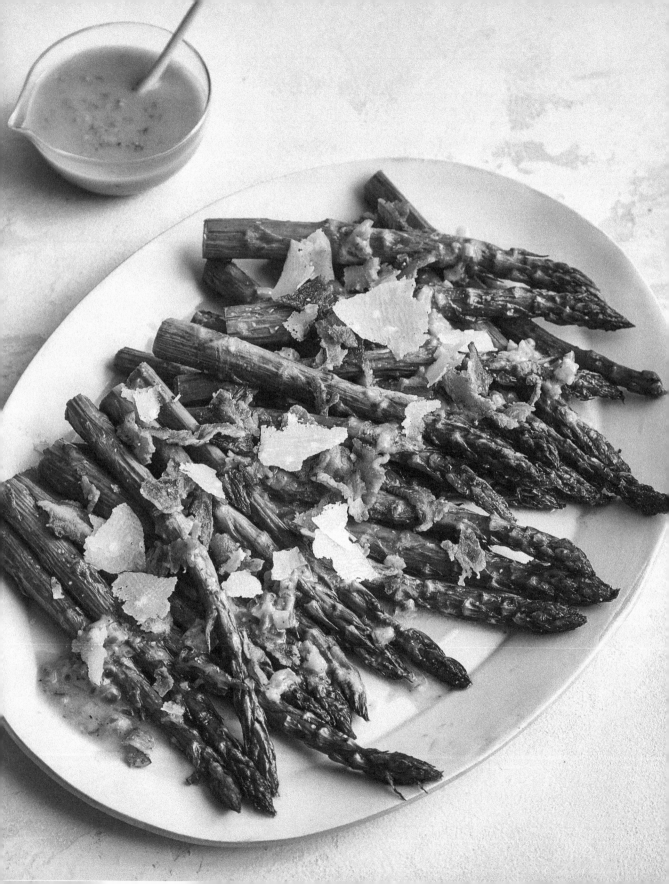

CHAPTER 5

Vegetables and Sides

Oven-Roasted Asparagus with Bacon Vinaigrette, page 82

Sheet Pan Garlic-and-Sesame Broccoli

Prep time: 10 minutes Cook time: 20 minutes

Roasting is one of my favorite ways to cook broccoli. Those caramelized bits are so delicious, and it really couldn't be easier. This garlicky, Asian-inspired broccoli is seasoned with nutty sesame oil and gets a kick from sriracha. It's perfect to spice up your weeknight meals. Serve with Fried Cauliflower Rice (page 92) for a satisfying vegetarian meal. **Serves 6**

1½ tablespoons avocado oil

2 garlic cloves, finely chopped

2½ teaspoons sesame oil

1 tablespoon soy sauce or tamari

2 teaspoons sriracha

1½ teaspoons granulated 1:1 sweetener

2 heads broccoli, cut into florets (about 6 cups)

2 teaspoons toasted sesame seeds

1. Preheat the oven to 450°F. Line a large baking sheet with parchment paper.

2. In a small bowl, combine the avocado oil, garlic, sesame oil, soy sauce, sriracha, and sweetener.

3. Put the broccoli in a large bowl. Drizzle the mixture over the broccoli and toss to coat.

4. Spread the broccoli on the lined baking sheet and roast for 15 to 18 minutes, or until tender, stirring halfway through the cooking time. Sprinkle with the sesame seeds and serve.

Tip: It's easy to add protein to this dish. Halfway through the cooking time, add about 1½ pounds of peeled and deveined shrimp to the baking sheet with the broccoli and toss to combine. Continue to cook as directed.

Per Serving Calories: 87; Total Fat: 6g; Total Carbs: 8g; Fiber: 3g; Net Carbs: 4g; Protein: 3g; Macros: Fat 62%/ Protein 14%/Carbs 24%

Roasted Brussels Sprouts with Lemon Aioli

Prep time: 15 minutes Cook time: 30 minutes

Brussels sprouts are one of my all-time favorite vegetable sides, and they are even better topped with the creamy tartness of lemon aioli. Brussels sprouts are a great keto side dish because they are loaded with fiber, which will help keep you full longer. Try the lemon aioli on other vegetables or as a delicious topping for grilled fish. **Serves 4**

1 pound Brussels sprouts, stemmed and halved

3 tablespoons extra-virgin olive oil

1¼ teaspoons kosher salt, divided

½ teaspoon freshly ground black pepper

½ cup keto-friendly mayonnaise or Three-Minute Mayo (page 178)

2 garlic cloves, minced

Grated zest of ½ lemon

1 tablespoon freshly squeezed lemon juice

1. Preheat the oven to 450°F.

2. In a medium bowl, toss together the Brussels sprouts, olive oil, 1 teaspoon salt, and the pepper.

3. Spread the Brussels sprouts on a large baking sheet and bake for 20 to 30 minutes, or until browned and tender, turning halfway through.

4. Meanwhile, in a small bowl, combine the mayonnaise, garlic, lemon zest, lemon juice, and remaining ¼ teaspoon salt.

5. As soon as the Brussels sprouts are cooked, put them in a medium bowl, spoon on half of the aioli, and toss. Serve with the remaining aioli on the side.

Tip: For an added kick, swap out the garlic for a little chili powder.

Per Serving Calories: 345; Total Fat: 33g; Total Carbs: 12g; Fiber: 5g; Net Carbs: 7g; Protein: 5g; Macros: Fat 86%/ Protein 6%/Carbs 8%

Oven-Roasted Asparagus with Bacon Vinaigrette

Prep time: 5 minutes Cook time: 15 minutes

Asparagus is delicious when roasted, and it take just minutes to cook it to crispy perfection. This recipe is dressed to impress with a bold, tangy vinaigrette, crispy bacon, and shaved Parmesan. **Serves 4**

1 pound asparagus, trimmed

3 tablespoons extra-virgin olive oil, divided

½ teaspoon kosher salt

¼ teaspoon freshly ground black pepper

4 bacon slices, diced

2 tablespoons finely diced red onion or shallot

1 garlic clove, finely minced

1½ tablespoons Dijon mustard

2 tablespoons red wine vinegar

2 ounces shaved Parmesan cheese

1. Preheat the oven to 425°F. Line a large baking sheet with parchment paper.

2. Place the asparagus on the baking sheet. Drizzle evenly with 1 tablespoon olive oil and season with the salt and pepper. Toss the asparagus spears to evenly coat and arrange them in a single layer. Roast for 10 to 15 minutes, or until tender and the tips of the spears begin to brown and crisp. If you are using asparagus with thicker spears, this may take a few minutes longer.

3. Meanwhile, prepare the vinaigrette. Heat a medium skillet over medium heat and cook the bacon until it's golden brown and crispy, 5 to 7 minutes. Remove the bacon from the pan and drain on a paper towel–lined plate. Pour off all but 3 tablespoons of bacon fat from the skillet.

4. Add the onion to the reserved bacon fat and sauté for 2 minutes over medium heat. Add the garlic and cook for another minute, then remove from the heat. Whisk in the Dijon mustard, vinegar, and remaining 2 tablespoons olive oil. Taste and season with salt and pepper as desired.

5. To serve, place the roasted asparagus on a serving plate, drizzle with the warm vinaigrette, sprinkle the crispy bacon over the asparagus, and top with the shaved Parmesan cheese.

Per Serving Calories: 217; Total Fat: 18g; Total Carbs: 6g; Fiber: 3g; Net Carbs: 3g; Protein: 8g; Macros: Fat 75%/Protein 15%/Carbs 10%

Elote-Style Grilled Cauliflower

Prep time: 5 minutes Cook time: 25 minutes

A popular street food in Mexico, elote is grilled corn on the cob that's smothered in a creamy mayo sauce called crema, sprinkled with cheese, and seasoned with chili and lime. This grilled (or roasted) cauliflower variation is dressed up with all the goodness of street corn, with a fraction of the carbs. It's a recipe you'll be making on repeat. **Serves 6**

1 large head cauliflower, cut into florets

3 tablespoons extra-virgin olive oil

¾ teaspoon kosher salt, divided

¾ teaspoon chili powder, divided

¼ teaspoon paprika

½ teaspoon garlic powder

¼ cup keto-friendly mayonnaise or Three-Minute Mayo (page 178)

¼ cup sour cream

¼ teaspoon ground cumin

1 or 2 garlic cloves, finely minced

2 teaspoons freshly squeezed lime juice

⅓ cup crumbled cotija cheese

2 tablespoons chopped fresh cilantro

1. To cook your cauliflower on the grill, preheat the grill to 425°F. Place the cauliflower florets in a disposable aluminum pan. Drizzle with the olive oil and season with ½ teaspoon salt, ½ teaspoon chili powder, the paprika, and garlic powder. Toss to coat.

2. Place the pan on the grill, cover, and cook for 20 to 25 minutes, stirring occasionally, until the cauliflower is tender and has started to char.

3. To cook your cauliflower in the oven, preheat the oven to 425°F. Line a large baking sheet with parchment paper. Place the cauliflower florets on the pan, drizzle with the olive oil, and season with ½ teaspoon salt, ½ teaspoon chili powder, the paprika, and garlic powder. Toss to coat.

4. Roast, stirring occasionally, for about 20 minutes, or until the florets are tender and golden brown.

5. Meanwhile, prepare the crema. In a small bowl, combine the mayonnaise, sour cream, remaining ¼ teaspoon salt, remaining ¼ teaspoon chili powder, the cumin, minced garlic, and lime juice.

6. Place the cooked cauliflower on a platter, drizzle with the prepared crema, and top with the cotija cheese and chopped cilantro.

Tip: Cotija cheese can be found in the specialty cheese section in many grocery stores. If you can't find it, crumbled feta makes the perfect substitute.

Per Serving Calories: 203; Total Fat: 19g; Total Carbs: 8g; Fiber: 3g; Net Carbs: 5g; Protein: 5g; Macros: Fat 84%/ Protein 10%/Carbs 6%

Sautéed Summer Squash

Prep time: 5 minutes Cook time: 10 minutes

Summer squash is a no-brainer when you're eating keto—especially because of its versatility. You can eat it sliced, chopped, or spiralized. Plus, its flavor is mild enough that you can mix and match seasonings. Feel free to add different spices to this super-simple dish to make it your own. **Serves 4**

3 tablespoons avocado oil

2 zucchini, halved lengthwise and cut into half-moons

2 yellow summer squash, halved lengthwise and cut into half-moons

Kosher salt

Freshly ground black pepper

4 teaspoons grated Parmesan cheese (optional)

1. In a large skillet, heat the avocado oil over medium heat.

2. Add the zucchini and yellow squash in as even a layer as possible. It should sizzle as it hits the skillet. Season with salt and pepper. Let the squash sit without stirring or moving for about 2 minutes, so it can get nice and golden on the bottom. After 2 minutes, give it a good stir and continue to cook for an additional 5 minutes, stirring occasionally, until the squash is tender.

3. Transfer to a bowl and sprinkle with the Parmesan cheese (if using).

Per Serving Calories: 124; Total Fat: 11g; Total Carbs: 6g; Fiber: 2g; Net Carbs: 4g; Protein: 2g; Macros: Fat 80%/Protein 6%/Carbs 14%

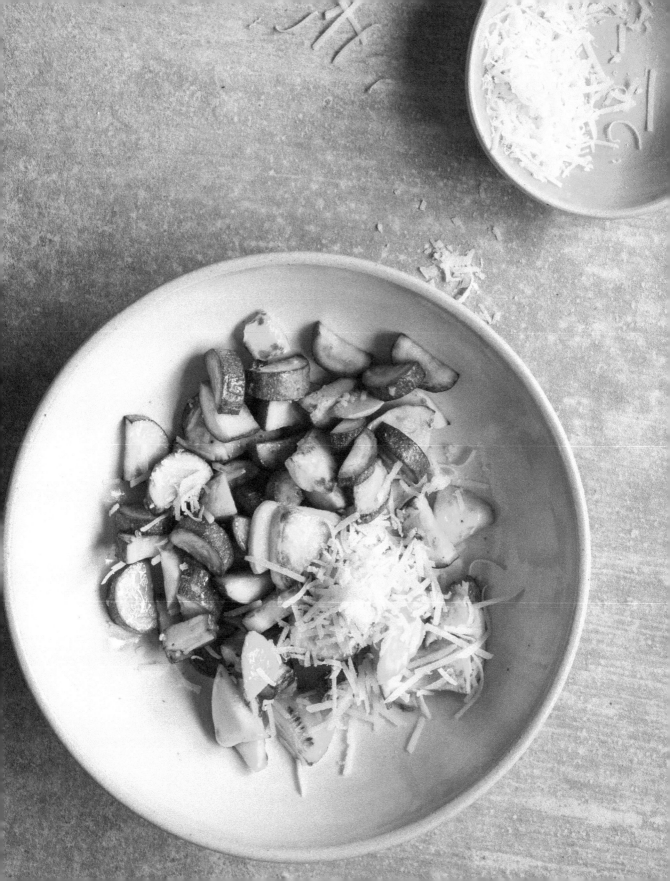

Creamed Spinach

Prep time: 10 minutes Cook time: 10 minutes

Fresh baby spinach is so versatile, so I always have it in the refrigerator. Use it as a quick base for a green salad, a healthy addition to a morning smoothie, or a topping for a burger, or cook it up in this super quick Creamed Spinach recipe. It goes perfectly with Crispy Chicken Thighs (page 117) or Parmesan-Crusted Baked Fish (page 111). **Serves 4**

4 tablespoons (½ stick) butter

½ cup diced onion

2 garlic cloves, finely chopped

1 pound baby spinach

½ teaspoon kosher salt

¼ teaspoon freshly ground black pepper

¼ cup heavy (whipping) cream

⅓ cup sour cream

1. In a large skillet, melt the butter over medium-high heat. Add the onion and sauté until tender, about 5 minutes. Add the garlic and cook for another minute.

2. Add the spinach to the pan, season with the salt and pepper, and sauté for 3 to 5 minutes, or until the spinach is wilted and tender.

3. Reduce the heat to low and stir in the heavy cream and sour cream. Cook until thoroughly heated.

Tip: For delicious, dairy-free, garlicky sautéed spinach, omit the heavy cream and sour cream. You can also omit the sour cream and substitute full-fat coconut milk or coconut cream for the heavy cream.

Per Serving Calories: 228; Total Fat: 21g; Total Carbs: 8g; Fiber: 3g; Net Carbs: 5g; Protein: 5g; Macros: Fat 83%/ Protein 9%/Carbs 8%

Zucchini-Parmesan Fritters

Prep time: 10 minutes Cook time: 10 minutes

These cheesy fritters are perfect served as a side with a grilled steak, but they are also just as delicious topped with smoked salmon and a dollop of sour cream for breakfast or a weekend brunch. **Serves 8**

2 medium zucchini, shredded (about 2 cups)

½ teaspoon kosher salt

½ cup grated Parmesan cheese

½ cup shredded mozzarella cheese

½ teaspoon granulated garlic

1 tablespoon chopped fresh parsley

½ teaspoon dried basil

3 tablespoons coconut flour

½ teaspoon baking powder

¼ teaspoon freshly ground black pepper

1 scallion, both white and light green parts, sliced

2 eggs, slightly beaten

2 tablespoons avocado oil

1. Place the shredded zucchini in a colander, toss with the salt, and let sit for 5 minutes. Squeeze the liquid from the zucchini, then place between two layers of paper towels and press to remove as much moisture as possible.

2. In a large mixing bowl, combine the drained zucchini, Parmesan cheese, mozzarella cheese, garlic, parsley, basil, coconut flour, baking powder, pepper, scallion, and eggs and stir until well mixed.

3. Line a plate with paper towels. In a large skillet, heat the avocado oil over medium-low to medium heat. Using a ¼-cup measuring cup, scoop up the mixture and use your hands to form it into patties. Place the patties in the pan and cook until lightly browned, 2 to 3 minutes per side.

4. Place the cooked fritters on the paper towel–lined plate to drain and repeat until all the zucchini mixture is used. Serve immediately.

Per Serving Calories: 117; Total Fat: 9g; Total Carbs: 5g; Fiber: 2g; Net Carbs: 3g; Protein: 6g; Macros: Fat 69%/Protein 21%/Carbs 10%

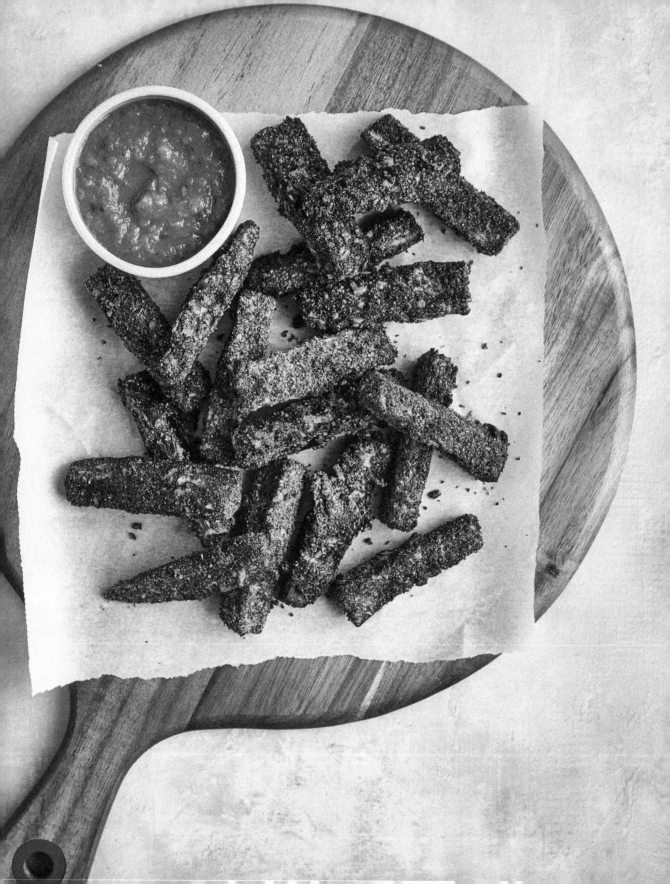

Eggplant Fries

Prep time: 10 minutes Cook time: 20 minutes

If you're missing French fries, these baked eggplant fries are a satisfying and delicious low-carb side to serve with a bunless burger or grilled steak. Dip them in Quick Marinara Sauce (page 183), or Three-Minute Mayo (page 178), or your favorite sugar-free ketchup. **Serves 6**

1½ tablespoons avocado oil

1 medium eggplant

½ cup ground flaxseed

½ cup grated Parmesan cheese

1 teaspoon Italian seasoning

½ teaspoon granulated garlic

½ teaspoon kosher salt

¼ teaspoon freshly ground black pepper

2 eggs

1. Preheat the oven to 450°F. Line a baking sheet with parchment paper and brush the parchment with the avocado oil. Set aside.

2. Remove the ends of the eggplant and cut lengthwise into ½-inch pieces, then cut into ½-inch sticks.

3. In a shallow dish or pie plate, combine the flax-seed, Parmesan cheese, Italian seasoning, garlic, salt, and pepper. In another dish, beat the eggs.

4. Dip the eggplant sticks into the beaten egg, then coat with the Parmesan cheese mixture. Place the coated sticks on the prepared baking sheet.

5. Bake for 15 to 20 minutes, or until golden, flip-ping over once halfway through cooking. Serve immediately.

Tip: If you're not a fan of eggplant, substitute zucchini for equally delicious keto-friendly fries.

Per Serving Calories: 166; Total Fat: 12g; Total Carbs: 10g; Fiber: 6g; Net Carbs: 4g; Protein: 8g; Macros: Fat 65%/Protein 19%/Carbs 16%

Fried Cauliflower Rice

Prep time: 5 minutes Cook time: 10 minutes

Chinese food is one of my take-out favorites, but it can be difficult to find keto-friendly options on the menu. So I started making some of the dishes at home. This easy fried "rice" can be on the table lightning fast and is extremely versatile. Serve it topped with Sheet Pan Garlic-and-Sesame Broccoli (page 80) for a meatless keto meal, or pair it with Sesame Chicken Kebabs (page 124). **Serves 4**

2 tablespoons avocado oil or coconut oil

3 garlic cloves, finely minced

2 scallions, both white and green parts, sliced

3 cups frozen cauliflower rice, thawed

1 egg, beaten

2 teaspoons sesame oil

3 tablespoons soy sauce, tamari, or coconut aminos

1. In a large skillet, heat the avocado oil over medium-high heat. Add the garlic and scallions and cook for about 1 minute. Add the cauliflower rice to the skillet and stir constantly until all the liquid is evaporated and the cauliflower begins to brown, 4 to 5 minutes

2. Reduce the heat to medium. Move the cauliflower rice to one side of the pan and add the beaten egg to the opposite side, stirring to scramble the egg. When the egg is almost cooked completely, stir together the egg and cauliflower.

3. Add the sesame oil and soy sauce and stir to combine. Serve immediately.

Tip: Add leftover steak, chicken, or even frozen shrimp for a fast keto dinner.

Per Serving Calories: 132; Total Fat: 10g; Total Carbs: 5g; Fiber: 2g; Net Carbs: 3g; Protein: 4g; Macros: Fat 68%/ Protein 12%/Carbs 20%

Zucchini Gratin

Prep time: 10 minutes Cook time: 30 minutes

Quick and easy, this cheesy zucchini gratin is one of the tastiest side dishes that will grace your dinner table. It's simple to make for a busy weeknight dinner and delicious enough for a special occasion or holiday dinner.

Serves 8

3 tablespoons butter

½ cup diced onion

1 teaspoon kosher salt, divided

2 garlic cloves, finely minced

4 zucchini, halved lengthwise and cut into half-moons

¾ cup heavy (whipping) cream

1½ cups shredded fontina, Gruyère, or Monterey Jack cheese, divided

½ teaspoon freshly ground black pepper

1. Preheat the oven to 400°F.

2. In a large oven-safe skillet, melt the butter over medium heat. Add the onion and season with ½ teaspoon salt. Cook until tender, about 5 minutes. Add the garlic and cook for another minute. Add the zucchini and season with the remaining ½ teaspoon salt. Sauté for about 5 minutes, or until the zucchini is just tender.

3. Stir in the heavy cream and cook for another minute, or until the sauce thickens. Remove from the heat and stir in 1 cup cheese. Mix to melt the cheese and form a creamy sauce.

4. Top with the remaining ½ cup cheese and bake for 10 to 12 minutes, or until the dish is bubbly. Turn the broiler on high and broil for 2 to 3 minutes, or until the top is browned.

5. Remove from the oven and let sit for 5 minutes before serving.

Per Serving Calories: 212; Total Fat: 19g; Total Carbs: 5g; Fiber: 1g; Net Carbs: 4g; Protein: 7g; Macros: Fat 81%/Protein 13%/Carbs 6%

Green Chile Cauliflower "Mac" and Cheese

Prep time: 10 minutes Cook time: 25 minutes

This version of cauliflower mac and cheese was inspired by a wildly delicious green chile mac and cheese my family loves at a barbecue place in a town. When we went keto, I had to come up with a tasty low-carb version to satisfy my family. To keep this side dish keto, cauliflower takes the place of traditional pasta and is paired with a quick and creamy green chile–Monterey Jack cheese sauce. **Serves 6**

Nonstick cooking spray

½ teaspoon kosher salt, plus more for boiling water

6 cups cauliflower florets

¾ cup heavy (whipping) cream

4 ounces cream cheese

¼ teaspoon granulated garlic

¼ teaspoon freshly ground black pepper

¼ teaspoon ground cumin

1½ cups shredded Monterey Jack cheese, divided

3 tablespoons canned diced mild green chiles

1. Preheat the oven to 350°F. Lightly grease a 9-inch square baking dish with cooking spray.

2. Fill a large stockpot or Dutch oven with water and a little salt and bring to a rolling boil. Add the cauliflower and cook for 6 to 9 minutes, or until it's fork-tender or at your preferred doneness. Drain the cauliflower well and let sit in the colander while you prepare the cheese sauce.

3. In a medium saucepan over medium heat, combine the heavy cream, cream cheese, salt, garlic, black pepper, and cumin. Bring the mixture to a simmer, then reduce the heat and simmer for 1 to 2 minutes. Remove from the heat and stir in 1 cup Monterey Jack cheese. Stir until the cheese is fully melted, then stir in the green chiles.

4. In a large bowl, combine the cheese sauce with the cauliflower and gently toss to coat the cauliflower.

5. Pour the cauliflower into the baking dish. Top with the remaining ½ cup Monterey Jack cheese and bake for 10 to 15 minutes, or until the cheese is melted.

Per Serving Calories: 301; Total Fat: 26g; Total Carbs: 8g; Fiber: 2g; Net Carbs: 6g; Protein: 11g; Macros: Fat 78%/ Protein 15%/Carbs 7%

Creamy Cabbage Alfredo

Prep time: 10 minutes Cook time: 15 minutes

You may think creamy, dreamy Alfredo sauce only belongs on pasta, but this quick cabbage Alfredo will change your mind after one bite. It's ridiculously addictive! This easy side comes together in one skillet in just minutes. Serve as a vegetarian main dish or dress it up with grilled shrimp, chicken, or steak. **Serves 8**

4 tablespoons
(½ stick) butter

1 (2½-pound) head green cabbage, cored and finely sliced

1½ teaspoons kosher salt

1 teaspoon freshly ground black pepper

1 teaspoon garlic powder

¼ cup cream cheese

¾ cup heavy (whipping) cream

¼ cup grated Parmesan cheese

1. In a large skillet, melt the butter over medium heat. Add the cabbage, season with the salt, pepper, and garlic powder, and sauté for 7 to 10 minutes, or until tender.

2. Reduce the heat to low and add the cream cheese, heavy cream, and Parmesan cheese. Stir until the cream cheese melts and the cabbage is coated with the sauce. Serve immediately.

Per Serving Calories: 195; Total Fat: 17g; Total Carbs: 8g; Fiber: 3g; Net Carbs: 5g; Protein: 4g; Macros: Fat 78%/ Protein 8%/Carbs 14%

Loaded Cauliflower Mash

Prep time: 15 minutes Cook time: 30 minutes

You won't miss mashed potatoes after you try this cauliflower mash. It's an especially stellar recipe to make when hosting non-keto guests. **Serves 10**

3 tablespoons unsalted butter, plus more for greasing

2 heads cauliflower, cut into small florets

6 bacon slices

4 ounces cream cheese, at room temperature

2½ cups shredded cheddar cheese, divided

2 tablespoons finely chopped fresh chives

2 teaspoons kosher salt

1 teaspoon garlic powder

½ teaspoon freshly ground black pepper

1. Preheat the oven to 450°F. Grease a 9-by-13-inch casserole dish with butter.

2. Fill a large stockpot halfway with water and bring to a boil over high heat. Once it's boiling, add the cauliflower. Boil until the cauliflower is fork-tender, about 15 minutes. Remove from the heat and drain the cauliflower.

3. Meanwhile, in a large pan, cook the bacon over medium heat to the desired level of crispiness, 8 to 12 minutes. Drain on a paper towel–lined plate, then crumble.

4. Using a food processor (or an immersion blender or potato masher), mash the cauliflower, cream cheese, and butter until the consistency is creamy. Add 1½ cups cheddar cheese, the chives, salt, garlic powder, and pepper and mix until combined. Spoon the cauliflower mixture into the casserole dish. Top with the remaining 1 cup cheese and the bacon crumbles.

5. Bake until the cheese is melted and starting to brown, about 15 minutes, and serve.

Per Serving Calories: 237; Total Fat: 19g; Total Carbs: 8g; Fiber: 2g; Net Carbs: 6g; Protein: 11g; Macros: Fat 72%/ Protein 19%/Carbs 9%

Pan-Roasted Red Radish "Potatoes"

Prep time: 10 minutes Cook time: 40 minutes

Roasted radishes are a delicious alternative to roasted red-skin potatoes. The moment you roast or boil them, radishes turn into warm, mild root vegetables that could almost be mistaken for potatoes in both texture and flavor. I use bacon fat in this recipe for maximum flavor, but olive oil or even melted butter are also good options. Enjoy these "potatoes" with any meat recipe. **Serves 6**

2 pounds red radishes, trimmed and halved

2 tablespoons melted bacon fat or extra-virgin olive oil

1 teaspoon kosher salt

½ teaspoon freshly ground black pepper

½ teaspoon garlic powder

½ teaspoon onion powder

½ teaspoon red pepper flakes (optional)

½ teaspoon Italian seasoning (optional)

1. Preheat the oven to 400°F. Line a large baking sheet with aluminum foil.

2. Spread the radishes on the baking sheet. Drizzle with the bacon fat. Sprinkle with the salt, black pepper, garlic powder, onion powder, red pepper flakes (if using), and Italian seasoning (if using) and toss to coat. Spread out in a single layer.

3. Bake on the center oven rack for 30 to 40 minutes (depending on the size of the radishes), or until golden brown and crispy. Toss halfway through cooking. When done, a fork should easily pierce the radishes.

Tip: If you ever see daikon radishes in your store and they're reasonably priced, pick some up. These long, bright-white radishes have a very mild flavor, and when sliced thick and roasted, they're a convincing potato alternative. They're a great substitute for the red radishes in this recipe.

Per Serving Calories: 65; Total Fat: 4g; Total Carbs: 6g; Fiber: 3g; Net Carbs: 3g; Protein: 1g; Macros: Fat 55%/ Protein 6%/Carbs 39%

Garlic-Cheddar Biscuits

Prep time: 5 minutes Cook time: 20 minutes

Who can resist warm, buttery biscuits? These garlic-cheddar biscuits satisfy cravings, and you'll avoid all the extra carbs. **Makes 10 biscuits**

1¾ cups shredded mozzarella cheese

¾ cup almond flour

2 tablespoons cream cheese

1 egg

¼ cup shredded cheddar cheese

2 teaspoons Italian seasoning

1 teaspoon onion powder

1 teaspoon kosher salt

4 tablespoons (½ stick) unsalted butter

1 tablespoon minced garlic

1 teaspoon kosher salt

½ teaspoon freshly ground black pepper

¼ cup grated Parmesan cheese

1. Preheat the oven to 350°F. Line a baking sheet with parchment paper.

2. In a large microwave-safe bowl, combine the mozzarella cheese, almond flour, and cream cheese and heat for 1½ minutes. Stir the mixture and return it to the microwave for an additional 1 minute.

3. Remove from the microwave and add the egg, cheddar cheese, Italian seasoning, onion powder, and salt and stir until well combined.

4. Drop the dough in 10 mounds (about 2 tablespoons each) onto the baking sheet. Bake for about 15 minutes, or until golden brown.

5. Melt the butter in a small microwave-safe bowl. Add the garlic, salt, and pepper.

6. Brush the biscuits with the butter mixture. Top them with the Parmesan cheese and serve.

Per Serving (1 biscuit) Calories: 193; Total Fat: 17g; Total Carbs: 3g; Fiber: 1g; Net Carbs: 2g; Protein: 8g; Macros: Fat 79%/Protein 17%/Carbs 4%

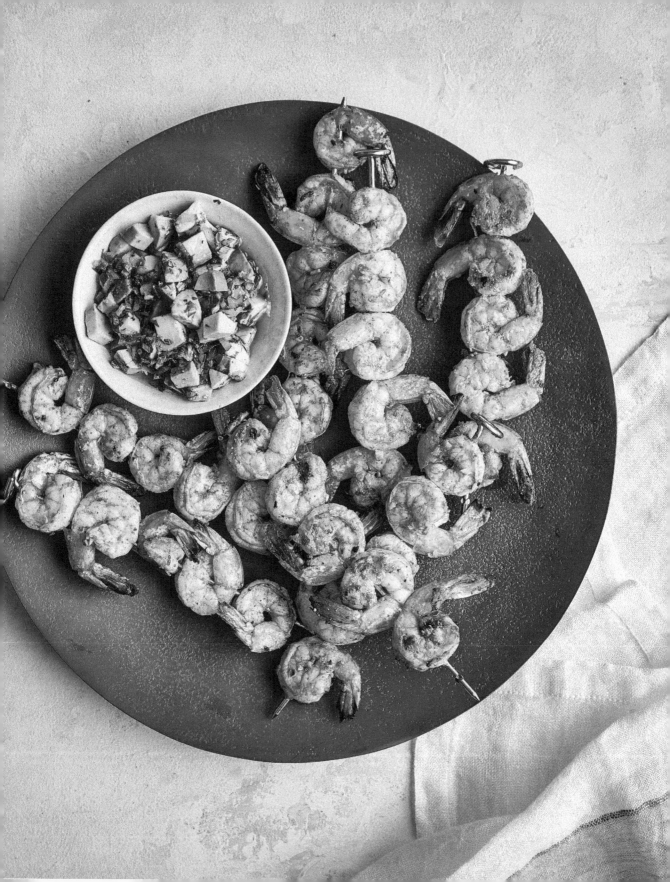

CHAPTER 6

Seafood and Chicken

Grilled Shrimp with Avocado Salsa, page 110

Bang Bang Shrimp

Prep time: 15 minutes Cook time: 5 minutes

These crispy, spicy shrimp cook up in just minutes. They're scrumptious served in a lettuce wrap, over Asian-Inspired Chopped Salad (page 64), over Fried Cauliflower Rice (page 92), or all on their own. **Serves 4**

½ cup keto-friendly mayonnaise or Three-Minute Mayo (page 178)

2 teaspoons sriracha

1 garlic clove, grated

½ teaspoon granulated 1:1 sweetener

½ teaspoon soy sauce or coconut aminos

½ teaspoon grated fresh ginger

½ teaspoon rice vinegar

1 pound large shrimp, peeled and deveined

⅓ cup unflavored whey protein isolate powder

¼ cup almond flour

½ cup grated Parmesan cheese

½ teaspoon granulated garlic

1 teaspoon kosher salt

½ teaspoon freshly ground black pepper

Avocado oil, for frying

2 eggs, beaten

1. In a small bowl, stir together the mayonnaise, sriracha, grated garlic, sweetener, soy sauce, ginger, and vinegar. Cover and refrigerate.

2. Pat the shrimp dry with paper towels. In a shallow pan, combine the protein powder, almond flour, Parmesan cheese, granulated garlic, salt, and pepper.

3. In a skillet, heat about ¼ inch of avocado oil over medium heat. Dip the shrimp in the beaten egg, let any excess drip off, then lightly coat in the Parmesan cheese mixture. Slip each shrimp into the hot oil right after it is coated.

4. Fry the shrimp for 1 to 2 minutes per side, or until golden brown. Drain on a paper towel–lined plate. Serve the shrimp hot, drizzled with the sauce.

Tip: You can find whey protein with the health foods in many supermarkets, as well as in health food stores and online. It creates a crispy crust when used as a breading for low-carb fried foods. You can substitute coconut flour, but the shrimp will not be as crispy.

Per Serving Calories: 452; Total Fat: 33g; Total Carbs: 6g; Fiber: 1g; Net Carbs: 5g; Protein: 35g; Macros: Fat 66%/ Protein 31%/Carbs 3%

Easy Barbecue Shrimp

Prep time: 10 minutes Cook time: 20 minutes

These delicious, peppery shrimp bake right in their shells, soaking up all the goodness of the tasty sauce. The result is a deliciously addictive sheet pan meal. Fresh shrimp are always best, but frozen unpeeled shrimp work just as well; just thaw and dry them before cooking. **Serves 4**

1 large lemon, sliced

1 medium onion, cut into wedges

8 tablespoons (1 stick) butter, melted

4 garlic cloves, finely minced

3 tablespoons Worcestershire sauce

2 tablespoons sugar-free barbecue sauce

2 teaspoons lemon pepper

1 teaspoon paprika

½ teaspoon kosher salt

⅛ teaspoon cayenne pepper

3 bay leaves

2 pounds large shrimp, unpeeled

1. Preheat the oven to 400°F.

2. Spread the lemon slices and onion wedges evenly on a 11-by-17-inch baking sheet.

3. In a large bowl, combine the butter, garlic, Worcestershire sauce, barbecue sauce, lemon pepper, paprika, salt, cayenne pepper, and bay leaves. Toss the shrimp in the butter mixture to coat.

4. Spread the shrimp out evenly on the baking sheet over the onions and lemon, scraping the bowl for any remaining sauce.

5. Bake for 15 to 20 minutes, or until the shrimp are pink and slightly curled. Serve immediately.

Per Serving Calories: 386; Total Fat: 25g; Total Carbs: 7g; Fiber: <1g; Net Carbs: 7g; Protein: 31g; Macros: Fat 58%/ Protein 32%/Carbs 10%

Cajun Shrimp "Pasta"

Prep time: 15 minutes Cook time: 25 minutes

Savory blackened shrimp swimming in a spicy Cajun cream sauce, served with zucchini noodles—this keto dinner couldn't get any better. If you don't have a spiralizer, zucchini noodles can often be found in the produce section or in the frozen food section of the grocery store. **Serves 4**

2 medium zucchini, spiralized

½ teaspoon kosher salt

1 pound large shrimp, peeled and deveined

2 tablespoons blackening seasoning

2 tablespoons butter

1 cup chicken stock or bone broth

2 garlic cloves, finely chopped

1 cup heavy (whipping) cream

½ cup grated Parmesan cheese

¼ cup shredded Asiago cheese

¼ teaspoon freshly ground black pepper

¼ cup sliced scallions, both white and green parts

1. Place the zucchini noodles in a colander and toss with the salt. Let sit for 5 minutes. Remove the noodles from the colander and pat dry between paper towels. Set aside.

2. In a large bowl, toss the shrimp with the blackening seasoning.

3. In a large skillet, melt the butter over medium-high heat. When it starts to sizzle, add the shrimp in batches of 6 to 8 (they should all lie flat in the skillet). Cook the shrimp for about 2 minutes, then flip and cook for another 2 to 3 minutes. Remove the shrimp and place in a bowl. Repeat until all the shrimp are cooked. Set aside.

4. Reduce the heat to medium and pour the chicken stock into the skillet. Stir, scraping up all of the seasoned bits from the bottom of the pan. Add the garlic to the pan, bring to a simmer, and cook for 2 to 3 minutes. Add the heavy cream and simmer for another 2 to 3 minutes. The cream mixture will start to reduce and thicken and will lightly coat the back of a spoon.

5. Reduce the heat to low and stir in the Parmesan and Asiago cheeses and stir constantly until all the cheese melts. Add the pepper, then taste the sauce and add salt as needed. Return the shrimp to the pan and stir to coat with the sauce. Add the zucchini noodles and scallions and toss gently to combine. Serve immediately.

Per Serving Calories: 453; Total Fat: 35g; Total Carbs: 8g; Fiber: 1g; Net Carbs: 7g; Protein: 29g; Macros: Fat 70%/Protein 26%/Carbs 4%

Crawfish Étouffée

Prep time: 10 minutes Cook time: 30 minutes

Spicy and comforting, étouffée is a Cajun stew made with seafood and vegetables. Don't let the ingredient list deter you; this easy dinner will be on the table in no time. Serve this étouffée over steamed cauliflower rice or your favorite low-carb rice alternative. **Serves 4**

1 teaspoon paprika

1 teaspoon dried oregano

1 teaspoon dried thyme

¼ teaspoon cayenne pepper

½ teaspoon freshly ground black pepper

½ teaspoon kosher salt

4 tablespoons (½ stick) butter

1 cup diced celery

1 cup diced bell pepper

¾ cup diced onion

4 garlic cloves, finely chopped

1 cup shrimp or chicken stock

½ cup heavy (whipping) cream

2 pounds frozen crawfish tails with fat, thawed

6 tablespoons cream cheese, at room temperature

¼ cup sliced scallions, both white and green parts

1. In a small bowl, combine the paprika, oregano, thyme, cayenne pepper, black pepper, and salt and set aside.

2. In a large skillet, melt the butter over medium heat. Cook the butter, stirring occasionally, for 3 to 5 minutes, or until lightly browned. Add the celery, bell pepper, and onion and continue to cook until the onion is translucent and the vegetables start to brown, 5 to 7 minutes. Add the garlic and cook for another minute. Stir the spice mixture into the vegetables and cook for another minute.

3. Add the stock to the vegetable mixture and stir well to combine. Simmer, uncovered, for 6 to 8 minutes. Then stir in the heavy cream and continue to simmer for another 5 to 7 minutes, or until the mixture has thickened and will coat the back of a spoon.

4. Once the sauce has thickened, add the crawfish and cook for 2 to 3 minutes. Remove from the heat and stir in the cream cheese. Sprinkle the scallions over the top of the crawfish. Serve immediately.

Tip: If you're unable to find crawfish tails, substitute 2 pounds of peeled and deveined medium shrimp.

Per Serving Calories: 451; Total Fat: 32g; Total Carbs: 9g; Fiber: 2g; Net Carbs: 7g; Protein: 35g; Macros: Fat 64%/Protein 31%/Carbs 5%

Parmesan-Crusted Scallops with Garlic Spinach

Prep time: 10 minutes Cook time: 10 minutes

When dinner needs to be on the table in less than 30 minutes, scallops are a perfect choice. Seared scallops are delicious, but these crispy, Parmesan-crusted scallops are downright decadent and a great keto option. Pair them with fresh spinach that you cook in the same pan. Fresh or frozen scallops will work in this recipe. Just make sure the frozen ones are completely thawed and thoroughly dried. **Serves 4**

12 sea scallops (about 1 pound)

½ cup grated Parmesan cheese

½ teaspoon freshly ground black pepper, divided

¼ teaspoon granulated garlic

6 tablespoons (¾ stick) butter, divided

2 garlic cloves, finely chopped

1 pound baby spinach

½ teaspoon kosher salt

1. Rinse the scallops and place on a paper towel lined–plate to dry, pressing the tops to remove as much moisture as possible.

2. On a plate or in a shallow dish, combine the Parmesan cheese, ¼ teaspoon pepper, and granulated garlic. Press each scallop into the cheese mixture to coat both sides.

3. In a large skillet, melt 2 tablespoons butter over medium-high heat. Place half the scallops in the pan and sear for 2 to 3 minutes, or until golden. Turn the scallops and cook for another 2 to 3 minutes. Remove from the pan and place on a wire rack. Repeat with the remaining scallops.

4. When all the scallops are cooked, melt the remaining 4 tablespoons butter in the same pan over medium-high heat. Add the chopped garlic and cook for 20 to 30 seconds, then add the spinach.

5. Season with the salt and remaining ¼ teaspoon pepper and sauté until the spinach is wilted. Serve immediately, topped with the seared scallops.

Per Serving Calories: 303; Total Fat: 22g; Total Carbs: 8g; Fiber: 3g; Net Carbs: 5g; Protein: 21g; Macros: Fat 65%/ Protein 28%/Carbs 7%

Grilled Shrimp with Avocado Salsa

Prep time: 15 minutes Cook time: 5 minutes

When the weather is nice, I like to shut down the kitchen and take the cooking outside to the grill. (I've included indoor cooking instructions as well.) Shrimp are a delicious and quick grilling option for a light, protein-packed keto meal.
Serves 4

2 garlic cloves, finely minced

½ teaspoon ground cumin

½ teaspoon chili powder

½ teaspoon paprika

2 tablespoons freshly squeezed lime juice, divided

1½ teaspoons kosher salt, divided

4 tablespoons extra-virgin olive oil, divided

1 pound large shrimp, peeled and deveined

2 ripe avocados, peeled, pitted, and diced

1 tablespoon chopped fresh cilantro

2 tablespoons finely diced red onion

¼ teaspoon freshly ground black pepper

1. Preheat the grill to 425°F or preheat your broiler.

2. In a large bowl, combine the garlic, cumin, chili powder, paprika, 1 tablespoon lime juice, 1 teaspoon salt, and 2 tablespoons olive oil. Add the shrimp and toss to coat. Let sit for 5 to 10 minutes.

3. Meanwhile, in a medium bowl, combine the avocados, remaining 2 tablespoons olive oil, the cilantro, onion, remaining 1 tablespoon lime juice, remaining ½ teaspoon salt, and pepper and stir to combine.

4. Thread the marinated shrimp onto skewers. When the grill is hot, place the shrimp on the grill and cook for 2 to 3 minutes per side, or until the shrimp is cooked through. If using the oven, place the shrimp on a baking sheet and broil for 2 to 3 minutes per side.

5. Carefully remove the shrimp from the skewers (they will be hot) and top with the avocado salsa.

Tip: Bamboo skewers should be soaked for at least 30 minutes before cooking to prevent burning.

Per Serving Calories: 331; Total Fat: 25g; Total Carbs: 8g; Fiber: 5g; Net Carbs: 3g; Protein: 22g; Macros: Fat 68%/ Protein 27%/Carbs 5%

Parmesan-Crusted Baked Fish

Prep time: 10 minutes Cook time: 15 minutes

This is one of the easiest and most delicious fish recipes you will ever eat. The crust not only keeps the fish nice and juicy, but it is also super delish. Any white fish will work for this recipe, including mahi mahi, flounder, pollock, grouper, cod, and bass. When shopping for fish, look for fillets that are about ½ inch thick. **Serves 4**

4 (6- to 8-ounce) white fish fillets

Kosher salt

Freshly ground black pepper

⅓ cup keto-friendly mayonnaise or Three-Minute Mayo (page 178)

1 garlic clove, grated

1 teaspoon Worcestershire sauce

½ teaspoon hot sauce

1 tablespoon freshly squeezed lemon juice

½ teaspoon Old Bay seasoning

½ cup grated Parmesan cheese

2 scallions, both white and green parts, sliced

¼ cup pork rind crumbs or pork panko

1. Preheat the oven to 425°F. Line a baking sheet with parchment paper.

2. Dry the fish fillets with paper towels and lightly season with salt and pepper. Place them on the prepared baking sheet.

3. In a small bowl, stir together the mayonnaise, garlic, Worcestershire sauce, hot sauce, lemon juice, and Old Bay seasoning. Add the Parmesan cheese and scallions. Spread the mixture evenly over the tops of the fillets. Sprinkle 1 tablespoon pork rind crumbs over each fillet.

4. Bake the fish for 10 to 14 minutes, or until done and flaky. Then place the fillets under the broiler for 1 to 2 minutes to crisp up the topping.

Per Serving Calories: 319; Total Fat: 22g; Total Carbs: 3g; Fiber: <1g; Net Carbs: 3g; Protein: 26g; Macros: Fat 62%/ Protein 33%/Carbs 5%

Grilled Salmon with Cilantro-Lime Crema

Prep time: 15 minutes Cook time: 20 minutes

Salmon is an excellent keto-friendly protein source and is loaded with vitamins, minerals, and omega-3 fatty acids. This Tex Mex–spiced grilled salmon is full of flavor and is delicious served over mixed greens or fresh baby spinach as a light lunch or dinner. **Serves 4**

¼ cup sour cream

¼ cup keto-friendly mayonnaise or Three-Minute Mayo (page 178)

1 tablespoon freshly squeezed lime juice

1 tablespoon chopped fresh cilantro

1 garlic clove, finely minced

⅛ teaspoon ground cumin

1¼ teaspoons kosher salt, divided

1¼ teaspoons dried oregano, crushed

¾ teaspoon granulated garlic

½ teaspoon paprika

½ teaspoon chili powder

⅛ teaspoon cayenne pepper

1 (1½-pound) salmon fillet, cut into 4 pieces

2 tablespoons avocado oil

Lime wedges, for serving (optional)

1. In a small mixing bowl, stir together the sour cream, mayonnaise, lime juice, cilantro, minced garlic, cumin, and ¼ teaspoon salt. Cover and refrigerate until you're ready to serve.

2. Preheat the grill or oven to 400°F.

3. In a small bowl, combine the oregano, granulated garlic, paprika, chili powder, cayenne pepper, and remaining 1 teaspoon salt.

4. Drizzle the pieces of salmon with the avocado oil and liberally season both sides with the spice mixture.

5. To cook on the grill, place the salmon, skin-side down, on the hot grill. Cook for 7 to 8 minutes per side, or until the salmon is cooked the way you like and the skin is crispy.

6. To cook in the oven, line a baking sheet with parchment paper. Place the salmon, skin-side down, on the pan. Bake for 8 to 10 minutes, then flip and continue to cook for an additional 7 to 9 minutes, depending on the thickness of the fish. To crisp up the skin, broil the salmon, skin-side up, for 2 to 3 minutes more.

7. To serve, spoon or drizzle the crema over the grilled salmon and serve with lime wedges (if using).

Tip: Try to find salmon with the skin on. It not only protects the fish while cooking, which creates a juicy, succulent piece of salmon, but crispy skin is also delicious. And it is the part of the fish with the highest concentration of omega-3 fatty acids.

Per Serving: Calories: 373; Total Fat: 26g; Total Carbs: 2g; Fiber: <1g; Net Carbs: 2g; Protein: 34g; Macros: Fat 63%/ Protein 36%/Carbs 1%

Seared Tuna Steak with Sriracha Aioli

Prep time: 10 minutes, plus up to 1 hour to marinate Cook time: 5 minutes

This recipe takes just minutes to prepare, and it's full of umami flavor from the ginger, lime, and soy marinade. Serve over Fried Cauliflower Rice (page 92) or Asian-Inspired Chopped Salad (page 64), topped with this easy sriracha aioli. When shopping, look for tuna that's about 1½ inches thick. **Serves 4**

1 teaspoon grated fresh ginger

4 garlic cloves, grated, divided

6 tablespoons soy sauce or tamari

2 tablespoons freshly squeezed lime juice

4 teaspoons sesame oil

4 teaspoons granulated 1:1 sweetener

½ teaspoon kosher salt

4 (4- to 5-ounce) tuna steaks

2 tablespoons avocado oil

½ cup keto-friendly mayonnaise or Three-Minute Mayo (page 178)

4 teaspoons sriracha

1. In a large zip-top bag, combine the ginger, half of the garlic, the soy sauce, lime juice, sesame oil, sweetener, and salt and mix well. Pat the tuna steaks dry with paper towels and place inside the bag with the marinade. Seal the bag and shake well to coat. Let the tuna steaks marinate in the refrigerator for at least 15 minutes, or up to 1 hour.

2. Preheat a heavy nonstick skillet over medium-high heat. Pour in the avocado oil and sear the tuna steaks for 2 to 3 minutes per side (about 2 minutes for medium-rare and 3 minutes for medium). Let the steaks rest for about 5 minutes.

3. Meanwhile, prepare the sriracha aioli. Combine the mayonnaise, remaining garlic, and sriracha in a small bowl. Slice the tuna steaks and serve with the aioli.

Tip: If your tuna is frozen, thaw the steaks in the refrigerator overnight, remove from the packaging, and pat dry with paper towels before cooking.

Per Serving Calories: 482; Total Fat: 35g; Total Carbs: 8g; Fiber: <1g; Net Carbs: 4g; Protein: 40g; Macros: Fat 65%/Protein 33%/Carbs 2%

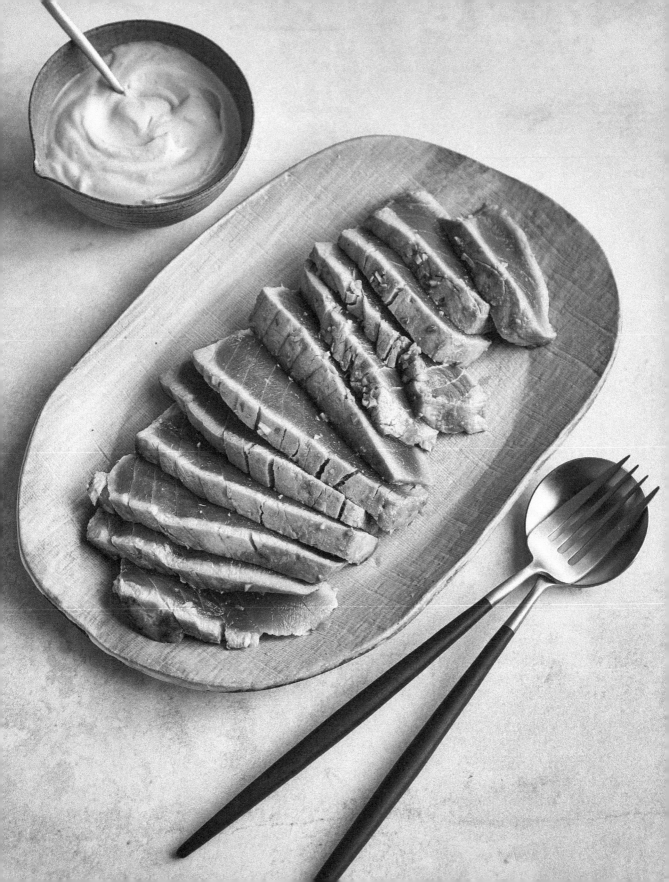

Creamy Seafood Stew

Prep time: 10 minutes Cook time: 35 minutes

This creamy chowder tastes authentic without having to buy budget-busting fresh seafood. By using canned shrimp, clams, and crab, you can achieve the same flavor at a fraction of the cost. **Serves 6**

8 ounces bacon, cut into 1-inch pieces

½ medium white onion, diced

2 celery stalks, diced

3 garlic cloves, minced

2 cups frozen cauliflower rice

1 teaspoon kosher salt

2 teaspoons freshly ground black pepper

3 cups low-sodium chicken stock

1 (8-ounce) bottle clam juice

1 (6-ounce) can medium shrimp, drained

1 (6-ounce) can crabmeat

1 (10-ounce) can chopped clams

1½ cups heavy (whipping) cream

8 ounces full-fat cream cheese, cubed, at room temperature

½ cup shredded cheddar cheese

1. In a large stockpot over medium heat, brown the bacon for 5 to 7 minutes, or until crispy. Remove to a paper towel–lined plate.

2. Pour off all but 2 tablespoons of bacon fat. Increase the heat to medium-high. Add the onion, celery, garlic, cauliflower rice, salt, and pepper. Sauté, stirring frequently, until the vegetables are soft, about 10 minutes.

3. Add the chicken stock and deglaze the pot with a wooden spoon. Reduce the heat to medium and simmer for 15 minutes.

4. Reduce the heat to low and add the clam juice, shrimp, crabmeat with its juices, and clams with their juices. Stir to combine. Add the heavy cream and cream cheese. Stir to melt the cream cheese and let sit, covered, on low heat for a few minutes to blend.

5. Serve in bowls, garnished with the bacon and cheddar cheese.

Per Serving Calories: 643; Total Fat: 52g; Total Carbs: 10g; Fiber: 1g; Net Carbs: 9g; Protein: 34g; Macros: Fat 73%/Protein 21%/Carbs 6%

Crispy Chicken Thighs

Prep time: 5 minutes, plus 2 to 4 hours to marinate Cook time: 50 minutes

With little to no cleanup, these simple chicken thighs will be a keto dinner staple. The cooking method is key here and ensures the skin on the thighs is crispy and delicious. Serve this juicy chicken with Creamed Spinach (page 88) or Creamy Cabbage Alfredo (page 96). **Serves 4**

8 bone-in, skin-on chicken thighs

¼ teaspoon onion powder

½ teaspoon granulated garlic

½ teaspoon paprika

½ teaspoon freshly ground black pepper, plus more as needed

1½ teaspoons kosher salt, plus more as needed

1½ tablespoons freshly squeezed lemon juice

1. Place the chicken thighs in a zip-top bag with the onion powder, garlic, paprika, pepper, salt, and lemon juice. Seal the bag, removing as much air as possible, and mix the seasoning with the chicken until it's evenly distributed. Refrigerate for 2 to 4 hours.

2. When you're ready to cook, remove the chicken from the bag and place on paper towels. Pat both sides of the chicken dry and season both sides of the chicken thighs lightly with salt and pepper.

3. Line a baking sheet with parchment paper and place the chicken on the pan, skin-side down. Put the pan in a cold oven and then turn it on to 425°F.

4. Roast the thighs for 25 minutes, then flip them over so the skin side is up. Roast for an additional 20 to 25 minutes, or until the chicken is fully cooked with an internal temperature of at least 165°F and the skin is golden brown and crispy. Serve immediately.

Per Serving Calories: 484; Total Fat: 38g; Total Carbs: 1g; Fiber: <1g; Net Carbs: <1g; Protein: 38g; Macros: Fat 70%/ Protein 30%/Carbs 0%

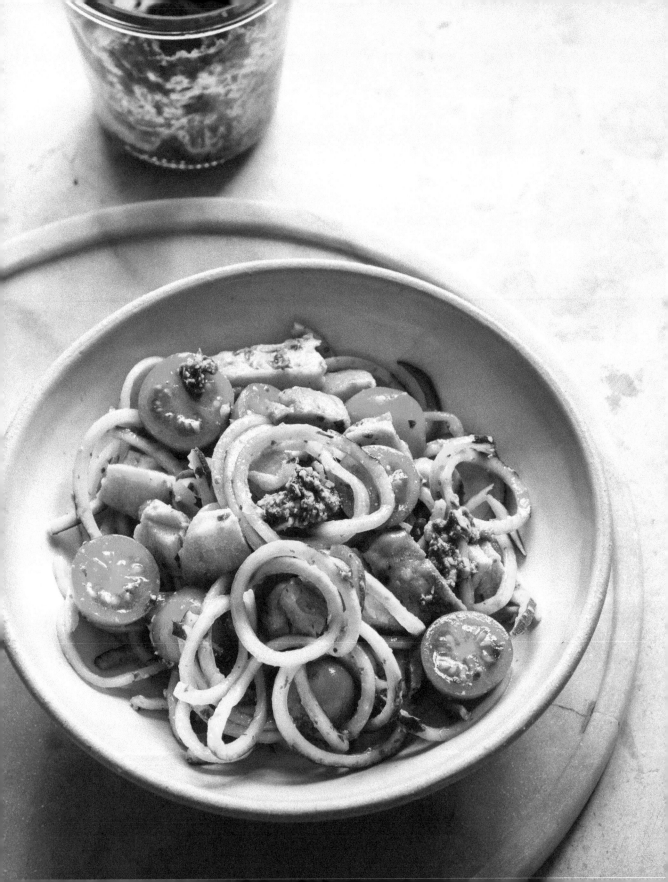

Chicken Zucchini "Pasta"

Prep time: 10 minutes Cook time: 10 minutes

This "pasta" is actually spiralized zucchini. It tastes great served warm or cold, which makes it extremely versatile. Be careful not to overcook the zucchini noodles, though—aim for an al dente texture. If you like, top it with some fresh mozzarella cheese. **Serves 4**

3 tablespoons butter or ghee

8 boneless, skinless chicken thighs, cubed

1 medium white onion, diced

6 garlic cloves, minced

2 zucchini, spiralized

4 teaspoons avocado oil

1 cup jarred pesto sauce

16 cherry tomatoes, halved

1. In a large skillet, melt the butter over medium-high heat. Add the chicken and onion and cook for several minutes, or until the chicken begins to brown. Add the garlic and cook for another 2 to 3 minutes, or until the chicken is cooked through. Reduce the heat to low.

2. In a medium bowl, coat the zucchini in the avocado oil. Add the zucchini to the skillet and cook for 1 minute, stirring occasionally.

3. Transfer the mixture to a medium bowl and toss with the pesto and tomatoes.

Tip: You can buy a spiralizer online for $20 to $30. But if you don't want one, look for packaged zucchini noodles in the produce section of the grocery store. Or, using a veggie peeler, peel the zucchini lengthwise into thin strips resembling noodles.

Per Serving Calories: 675; Total Fat: 54g; Total Carbs: 12g; Fiber: 3g; Net Carbs: 9g; Protein: 42g; Macros: Fat 72%/Protein 25%/Carbs 3%

Salsa Verde Chicken

Prep time: 5 minutes Cook time: 35 minutes

Forget Taco Tuesday. This quick and easy Mexican-inspired dish is an even better weeknight dinner. Because they're high in protein, chicken breasts will keep you full, which makes them ideal for keto, but they can be somewhat boring. This recipe amps things up with a creamy green tomatillo salsa and plenty of melty cheese. Serve it over steamed cauliflower rice or spaghetti squash, topped with a dollop of sour cream. **Serves 4**

2 tablespoons avocado oil, plus more for greasing

4 (4- to 6-ounce) boneless, skinless chicken breasts

¾ teaspoon kosher salt

½ teaspoon freshly ground black pepper

1 teaspoon granulated garlic

2 cups mild green salsa or enchilada sauce

⅓ cup heavy (whipping) cream

1½ cups grated Monterey Jack or pepper Jack cheese

1. Preheat the oven to 400°F. Lightly grease a 9- or 10-inch baking dish with avocado oil.

2. Drizzle the chicken breasts with the avocado oil and season with the salt, pepper, and garlic on both sides, then place the chicken breasts in the baking dish.

3. In a small bowl, stir together the salsa and heavy cream and pour over the chicken, making sure all the chicken is coated. Bake for about 25 minutes, or until the chicken is cooked through.

4. Evenly sprinkle the Monterey Jack cheese over the chicken and return to the oven for another 10 minutes, or until the cheese is melted and the internal temperature of the chicken is 165°F.

Tip: Opt for a hotter salsa or enchilada sauce to kick things up a notch.

Per Serving Calories: 456; Total Fat: 31g; Total Carbs: 9g; Fiber: 2g; Net Carbs: 7g; Protein: 37g; Macros: Fat 61%/ Protein 32%/Carbs 7%

Cheesy Artichoke Chicken

Prep time: 10 minutes Cook time: 25 minutes

If you love artichoke dip, this creamy casserole will be your new dinner obsession. Use leftover chicken to get this cheesy chicken dish on the table in just 30 minutes, and serve over steamed cauliflower rice or with a simple green salad. **Serves 4**

Nonstick cooking spray

2 cups shredded
cooked chicken

1 (14-ounce) can artichoke
hearts, drained and chopped

4 ounces cream cheese, at
room temperature

¼ cup keto-friendly
mayonnaise or Three-Minute
Mayo (page 178)

¼ cup sour cream

¼ cup heavy
(whipping) cream

¼ teaspoon
Worcestershire sauce

½ teaspoon hot sauce

½ teaspoon kosher salt

½ teaspoon freshly ground
black pepper

2 garlic cloves, finely minced

½ cup grated
Parmesan cheese

1 cup shredded fontina or
mozzarella cheese, divided

1. Preheat the oven to 375°F. Lightly grease a 9-inch square baking dish with cooking spray.

2. In a medium bowl, combine the chicken, artichokes, cream cheese, mayonnaise, sour cream, heavy cream, Worcestershire sauce, hot sauce, salt, pepper, garlic, Parmesan cheese, and ½ cup fontina cheese. Stir the mixture until completely combined.

3. Pour the chicken mixture into the prepared baking dish and spread evenly. Top with the remaining ½ cup fontina cheese and bake for 20 to 25 minutes, or until bubbly and golden brown.

Per Serving Calories: 651; Total Fat: 45g; Total Carbs: 14g; Fiber: 7g; Net Carbs: 7g; Protein: 38g; Macros: Fat 62%/ Protein 23%/Carbs 5%

One-Pan Chicken Parmesan

Prep time: 15 minutes Cook time: 25 minutes

Italian food is one of my weaknesses, and this easy chicken Parmesan is one of my cravings. Traditionally, the chicken cutlets are coated with bread crumbs, but in this keto version, Parmesan cheese creates the crust for the juicy chicken. It's then topped with marinara sauce and cheese, making one delicious keto meal. **Serves 4**

2 chicken breasts, halved horizontally to make 4 cutlets total

½ cup grated Parmesan cheese

½ teaspoon Italian seasoning

½ teaspoon granulated garlic

½ teaspoon freshly ground black pepper

3 tablespoons keto-friendly mayonnaise or Three-Minute Mayo (page 178)

1½ tablespoons avocado oil or extra-virgin olive oil

1½ cups sugar-free marinara sauce or Quick Marinara Sauce (page 183)

1½ cups shredded mozzarella or provolone cheese

1. Preheat the oven to 400°F.

2. Place each chicken cutlet between two sheets of plastic wrap and pound with a meat mallet or rolling pin to flatten to about ¼ inch thick.

3. In a shallow dish, combine the Parmesan cheese, Italian seasoning, garlic, and pepper. Brush each piece of chicken on both sides with the mayonnaise and coat lightly with the Parmesan cheese mixture.

4. In a large oven-safe skillet, heat the avocado oil over medium heat. Add the chicken and cook for 4 to 5 minutes on each side, until golden brown. Remove from the heat.

5. Pour the marinara sauce over the chicken and top with the mozzarella cheese. Bake for 10 to 15 minutes, or until the cheese is melted and the chicken is cooked through.

Per Serving Calories: 518; Total Fat: 33g; Total Carbs: 9g; Fiber: 2g; Net Carbs: 7g; Protein: 45g; Macros: Fat 57%/ Protein 35%/Carbs 8%

Lemon-Basil Grilled Chicken

Prep time: 10 minutes, plus 1 hour to marinate Cook time: 35 minutes

The classic combination of lemon and basil take these simple grilled chicken thighs to the next level. Use this flavorful chicken to top a green salad, fill a lettuce wrap, or provide a protein accompaniment to Zucchini Gratin (page 93). **Serves 4**

3 tablespoons freshly squeezed lemon juice

2 tablespoons chopped fresh basil

2 garlic cloves, minced

¼ cup avocado oil

8 boneless, skinless chicken thighs

2 teaspoons kosher salt

1 teaspoon freshly ground black pepper

1. In a blender or food processor, blend the lemon juice, basil, garlic, and avocado oil for 20 to 30 seconds. Reserve ¼ cup of the lemon-basil mixture and set aside.

2. Place the chicken thighs in a zip-top bag and add the remaining marinade. Seal the bag and refrigerate for 1 hour.

3. When you're ready to cook, preheat the grill or smoker to 375°F to 400°F. Remove the chicken from the bag and discard the marinade. Season the chicken thighs with the salt and pepper and grill for 30 to 35 minutes, or until the internal temperature reaches at least 160°F, basting with the reserved lemon-basil mixture while grilling.

Tip: To cook this dish in the oven, preheat the oven to 425°F. Place the chicken thighs on a baking sheet lined with parchment paper and roast for 25 to 35 minutes, or until the internal temperature reaches at least 160°F, turning once while cooking. Baste with the reserved lemon-basil mixture at least twice while cooking.

Per Serving Calories: 387; Total Fat: 28g; Total Carbs: 2g; Fiber: <1g; Net Carbs: <2g; Protein: 36g; Macros: Fat 65%/Protein 35%/Carbs 0%

Sesame Chicken Kebabs

Prep time: 10 minutes Cook time: 25 minutes

The sweet and sticky glaze that coats this juicy grilled chicken is possible thanks to the addition of allulose, a sweetener that doesn't crystallize when heated. Serve this over steamed cauliflower rice. **Serves 4**

⅓ cup soy sauce or coconut aminos

⅓ cup rice vinegar

¼ cup water

¼ cup granulated 1:1 allulose-based sweetener

½ teaspoon grated fresh ginger

1 garlic clove, smashed

½ teaspoon red pepper flakes

6 boneless, skinless chicken thighs, cut into 2-inch pieces

1 bell pepper, seeded and cut into 1½-inch pieces

2 medium zucchini, cut into ¾-inch pieces

1 small red onion, cut into 1½-inch pieces

2 teaspoons toasted sesame seeds

1. Preheat the grill to 375°F to 400°F. Or preheat the oven to 425°F and line a baking sheet with parchment paper.

2. In a small saucepan, combine the soy sauce, vinegar, water, sweetener, ginger, garlic, and red pepper flakes and bring to a boil. Cook for 5 to 6 minutes, or until the sauce is reduced and slightly thickened. Remove from the heat and set aside.

3. Meanwhile, thread the chicken onto skewers, folding the meat as needed and alternating with pieces of bell pepper, zucchini, and onion.

4. Grill the kebabs for 3 to 5 minutes per side, or until the chicken is done, basting with the glaze every few minutes. The kebabs will have char spots and be a mahogany color.

5. If you're cooking the kebabs in the oven, place them on the prepared baking sheet and roast for 15 to 20 minutes, rotating the kebabs and basting often with the glaze.

6. Remove the chicken from the grill or the oven, sprinkle with the toasted sesame seeds, and serve.

Per Serving Calories: 256; Total Fat: 12g; Total Carbs: 20g; Fiber: 2g; Net Carbs: 6g; Protein: 31g; Macros: Fat 42%/ Protein 48%/Carbs 10%

Cheesy Chicken-Broccoli Casserole

Prep time: 10 minutes Cook time: 30 minutes

This cheesy chicken casserole was inspired by one of my childhood favorites. No need to pop open any canned soups; a quicker and better version can be made with fresh veggies and cream. **Serves 6**

2 tablespoons butter, plus more for greasing

½ cup chopped celery

½ cup chopped white onion

½ cup chopped white mushrooms

2 teaspoons kosher salt, divided

3 cups frozen broccoli florets, thawed and roughly chopped

1 cup heavy (whipping) cream

4 ounces cream cheese

2½ cups shredded Colby Jack cheese

¾ cup sour cream

3 cups shredded cooked chicken

1 teaspoon freshly ground black pepper

½ teaspoon granulated garlic

1. Preheat the oven to 375°F. Grease a 9-by-13-inch baking pan with butter.

2. In a medium skillet, melt the butter over medium-high heat and add the celery, onion, and mushrooms. Season with 1 teaspoon salt and cook for about 5 minutes. Add the broccoli and cook for another 2 to 3 minutes, until heated through.

3. Reduce the heat to medium and add the heavy cream and cream cheese to the skillet. Stir constantly until the sauce is thick and creamy, 1 to 2 minutes.

4. In a large bowl, combine 1½ cups Colby Jack cheese, the sour cream, chicken, remaining 1 teaspoon salt, pepper, garlic, and cooked vegetable mixture with sauce and stir until combined.

5. Spread the mixture evenly in the prepared pan and top with the remaining 1 cup Colby Jack cheese. Bake for 15 to 20 minutes, or until hot and bubbly.

Per Serving Calories: 590; Total Fat: 47g; Total Carbs: 10g; Fiber: 3g; Net Carbs: 7g; Protein: 34g; Macros: Fat 72%/Protein 23%/Carbs 5%

Avocado-Chicken Burgers

Prep time: 5 minutes Cook time: 20 minutes

Possibly one of the healthiest and most satisfying dinner recipes for the keto diet is an avocado-chicken burger. Packed with healthy fats, avocado is the ultimate addition to any protein-based meal. Top these burgers with alfalfa sprouts and goat cheese, a slice of Swiss cheese, or any other favorite keto-friendly toppings. **Serves 4**

1 pound ground chicken

½ cup almond flour

2 garlic cloves, minced

1 teaspoon onion powder

¼ teaspoon kosher salt

⅛ teaspoon freshly ground black pepper

1 avocado, peeled, pitted, and diced

2 tablespoons extra-virgin olive oil

4 low-carb buns or lettuce wraps (optional)

1. In a large bowl, mix together the chicken, almond flour, garlic, onion powder, salt, and pepper. Add the avocado, gently incorporating it into the meat. Use your hands to form four patties.

2. In a large skillet, heat the olive oil over medium heat for about 1 minute. Add the patties to the skillet. Cook for about 8 minutes per side, or until golden brown and cooked through.

3. Serve on a low-carb bun (if using), in a lettuce wrap (if using), or on their own.

Tip: If topping your burger with alfalfa sprouts, it's important to remember that they can sometimes carry harmful bacteria. To avoid this problem, wash them a minimum of two times before eating.

Per Serving Calories: 363; Total Fat: 28g; Total Carbs: 7g; Fiber: 4g; Net Carbs: 3g; Protein: 23g; Macros: Fat 69%/ Protein 25%/Carbs 6%

White Chicken Chili

Prep time: 15 minutes Cook time: 35 minutes

When it's cold outside, there's nothing like a piping hot bowl of chili. This version will satisfy your cravings without the carbs. Serve topped with your favorite keto-friendly toppings. **Serves 6**

1 teaspoon extra-virgin olive oil, plus more for greasing

2 (6-ounce) boneless, skinless chicken breasts

1 tablespoon unsalted butter

½ onion, diced

2 garlic cloves, minced

2 cups chicken stock

1 (28-ounce) can diced tomatoes

6 tablespoons tomato paste

1 jalapeño pepper, diced

1 tablespoon chili powder

1 tablespoon ground cumin

1 tablespoon garlic powder

2 teaspoons kosher salt

1 teaspoon freshly ground black pepper

8 ounces cream cheese, cut into 1-inch chunks

1. In a large skillet, heat the olive oil over medium-high heat. Add the chicken breasts and cook for 6 to 8 minutes per side, or until the internal temperature reaches 165°F. Let the chicken rest for 5 minutes before shredding with two forks.

2. In a large stockpot, melt the butter over medium-high heat. Add the onion and minced garlic and cook until softened, about 5 minutes. Add the shredded chicken, chicken stock, diced tomatoes with their juices, tomato paste, jalapeño, chili powder, cumin, garlic powder, salt, and pepper and gently stir to combine.

3. Bring to a boil, then reduce the heat to medium-low, cover, and simmer until the flavors combine, about 10 minutes.

4. Add the cream cheese to the chili. Increase the heat to medium-high and stir until the cream cheese is incorporated.

Per Serving Calories: 295; Total Fat: 18g; Total Carbs: 16g; Fiber: 4g; Net Carbs: 12g; Protein: 19g; Macros: Fat 55%/ Protein 26%/Carbs 19%

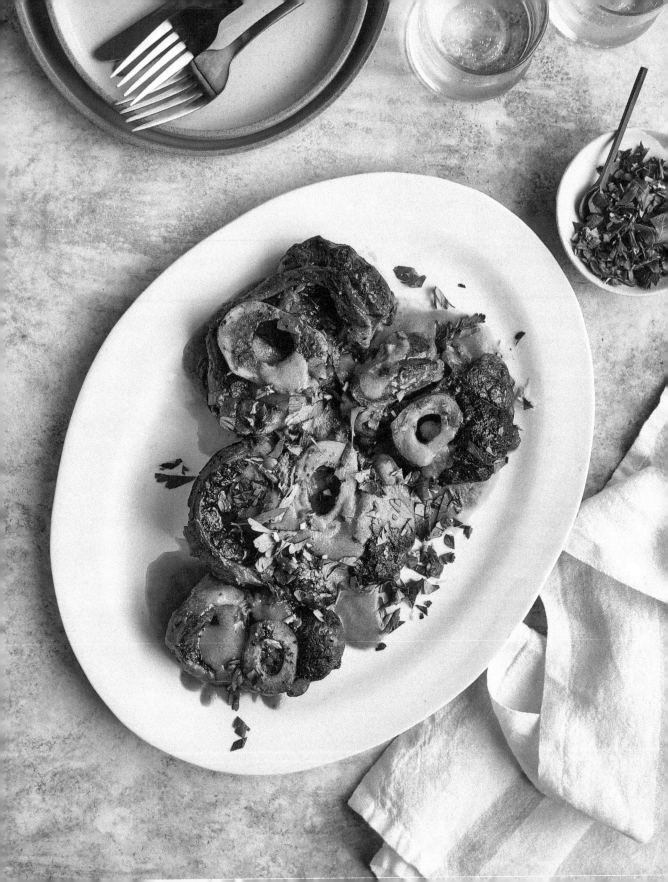

CHAPTER 7

Beef, Pork, and Lamb

Osso Bucco, page 140

Flank Steak with Avocado Butter

Prep time: 5 minutes Cook time: 5 minutes

Super flavorful and affordable, flank steak is one of my favorite cuts of beef. The secret to cooking a mouthwatering flank steaks is to sear it hot and quick and cut it thinly across the grain. Top it with Avocado Butter (page 180) and serve with Green Chile Cauliflower "Mac" and Cheese (page 94). **Serves 4**

1½ teaspoons kosher salt

1 teaspoon freshly ground black pepper

1 teaspoon granulated garlic

½ teaspoon paprika

½ teaspoon chili powder

½ teaspoon ground cumin

2 tablespoons butter, at room temperature

1½ pounds flank steak

Avocado Butter (page 180)

1. In a small bowl, combine the salt, pepper, garlic, paprika, chili powder, and cumin.

2. Rub 1 tablespoon butter evenly over one side of the steak, then sprinkle half of the seasoning over the butter. Repeat with the other side of the steak.

3. Heat a large, heavy-bottomed skillet over medium-high heat. Place the steak in the skillet and sear for 2 to 3 minutes per side, or until it's cooked the way you like. Remove the steak from the pan, cover with aluminum foil, and let rest for at least 5 minutes.

4. Slice thinly and serve topped with avocado butter.

Tip: To grill, heat to 400°F to 425°F. Omit the butter and brush the steak with avocado oil before seasoning. Place the steak on the grill, cover, and cook for 4 to 7 minutes on each side. Let the steak rest for at least 5 minutes before slicing.

Per Serving Calories: 357; Total Fat: 21g; Total Carbs: 2g; Fiber: 1g; Net Carbs: 1g; Protein: 36g; Macros: Fat 53%/ Protein 40%/Carbs 7%

Quick Skillet Stroganoff

Prep time: 5 minutes Cook time: 20 minutes

This creamy beef and mushroom dish is on our family's top 10 list. I make it with ground beef, since I almost always have some on hand, and it makes a super quick weeknight meal. **Serves 4**

3 tablespoons butter

½ cup diced onion

8 ounces mushrooms, sliced

1½ teaspoons kosher salt, divided

1 pound ground beef

2 teaspoons granulated garlic

1½ teaspoons paprika

½ teaspoon freshly ground black pepper

½ cup dry white wine, dry sherry, or beef stock

½ cup beef stock or bone broth

1 tablespoon tomato paste

1 (14-ounce) can hearts of palm pasta, drained and rinsed, or 2 cups cauliflower rice

¼ cup cream cheese, at room temperature

⅓ cup sour cream

1. In a large skillet, melt the butter over medium-high heat. Add the onion, mushrooms, and ½ teaspoon salt and sauté for about 5 minutes, or until the onions are translucent and the mushrooms are tender. Remove from the skillet and set aside.

2. In the same skillet, combine the ground beef, garlic, paprika, remaining 1 teaspoon salt, and the pepper. Cook the ground beef for 7 to 8 minutes, breaking it up with a wooden spoon, until browned.

3. Increase the heat to high, add the wine, and deglaze the pan, scraping up any browned bits from the bottom. Add the beef stock and tomato paste and stir to combine. Cook for another 1 to 2 minutes, until the liquid is reduced by half.

4. Reduce the heat to medium, then add the mushroom mixture and hearts of palm pasta. Stir until heated through. Add the cream cheese and sour cream and keep stirring until the cheese melts and everything is thoroughly combined and thickened. Serve immediately.

Per Serving Calories: 509; Total Fat: 36g; Total Carbs: 10g; Fiber: 3g; Net Carbs: 7g; Protein: 34g; Macros: Fat 64%/ Protein 27%/Carbs 9%

Italian-Style Shredded Beef

Prep time: 10 minutes Cook time: 4 hours

I love easy dishes like this that are quickly prepared on the stovetop, then go into the oven for a few hours. This makes great leftovers, as it's even better the next day. **Serves 6**

3 tablespoons avocado oil

1 (3- to 4-pound) boneless chuck roast

2 teaspoons kosher salt

1 teaspoon freshly ground black pepper

3 celery stalks, diced

1 small onion, diced

3 garlic cloves, minced

2 cups beef stock or bone broth

¾ cup sugar-free marinara or Quick Marinara Sauce (page 183)

2 bay leaves

½ teaspoon dried oregano

½ teaspoon dried basil

1. Preheat the oven to 325°F.

2. In a Dutch oven heat the avocado oil over medium-high heat. Season the roast with the salt and pepper and add to the pot. Brown on all sides, remove from the pot, and set aside.

3. Add the celery and onion to the pot and cook, stirring constantly, until the onion is tender, about 5 minutes. Add the garlic and cook for another minute. Deglaze the pan with the stock.

4. Add the marinara sauce, bay leaves, oregano, and basil, then return the roast to the pot. Bring the liquid to a boil, cover, and place the pot in the oven on the center rack. Roast for 3½ to 4 hours, or until tender.

5. Remove the roast from the pot and shred using two forks. Remove the bay leaves from the broth. Mix the shredded beef back into the pan juices and serve.

Per Serving Calories: 633; Total Fat: 46g; Total Carbs: 5g; Fiber: 1g; Net Carbs: 4g; Protein: 46g; Macros: Fat 65%/Protein 29%/Carbs 6%

Texas Goulash

Prep time: 5 minutes Cook time: 20 minutes

When I was growing up, my dad called any skillet meal made with ground meat and pasta "goulash," and it was always one of my comfort foods. This spiced-up version reminds me of the chili mac of my childhood. Serve this hearty dish topped with shredded cheese, sliced avocado, and a dollop of sour cream. **Serves 4**

1½ pounds ground beef

1 teaspoon kosher salt

½ cup diced onion

1 teaspoon granulated garlic

2 tablespoons chili powder

1 (7-ounce) package shirataki macaroni noodles, drained and rinsed

¾ cup chicken stock or bone broth

½ cup grated mild cheddar cheese

2 tablespoons grated Parmesan cheese

1. In a skillet over medium-high heat, brown the ground beef and season with the salt. When the meat is about halfway cooked, add the onions and continue to cook until the meat is completely browned and caramelized and the onions are translucent, 5 to 7 minutes.

2. Stir in the garlic, chili powder, and noodles and cook for another minute. Add the stock and cook for 3 to 4 minutes, or until the stock is reduced to about ⅓ cup.

3. Reduce the heat to low and stir in the cheddar and Parmesan cheeses. Continue to cook, stirring, for 1 to 2 minutes, or until the mixture thickens slightly. Serve immediately.

Tip: Feel free to use your favorite pasta alternative in place of the shirataki noodles in this hearty dish. Hearts of palm "pasta," leftover spaghetti squash, or zucchini noodles would all work well in this dish.

Per Serving Calories: 527; Total Fat: 34g; Total Carbs: 6g; Fiber: 3g; Net Carbs: 3g; Protein: 49g; Macros: Fat 58%/ Protein 37%/Carbs 5%

Garlic Steak Bites with Mushrooms and Asparagus

Prep time: 10 minutes Cook time: 15 minutes

Quick and easy, this steak dish is packed with flavor and can be on the table in less than 30 minutes. Other cuts of steak, such as strip, tenderloin, and rib eye, will also work for this recipe. **Serves 4**

1½ pounds sirloin steak, cut into 1-inch cubes

Kosher salt

Freshly ground black pepper

3 tablespoons avocado oil

3 tablespoons butter

8 ounces mushrooms, sliced

1 pound asparagus, trimmed and cut into 2-inch pieces

2 teaspoons minced garlic

1. Season the beef well with salt and pepper. In a large, heavy-bottomed skillet, heat the avocado oil over medium-high heat. When the oil is hot and begins to shimmer, add some of the beef cubes in a single layer without crowding the pan. Cook for about 1½ to 2 minutes, flipping each piece halfway through. Remove from the pan and repeat with the remaining beef.

2. Reduce the heat to medium and melt the butter in the pan. Add the mushrooms and cook for about 5 minutes. Use the mushrooms and any liquid they release to deglaze the pan, scraping up any browned bits from the bottom.

3. Add the asparagus pieces and cook for another 5 to 6 minutes, stirring often, until the asparagus is tender. Add the garlic and cook for another minute. Return the beef to the pan and toss to combine. Serve immediately.

Per Serving Calories: 434; Total Fat: 27g; Total Carbs: 7g; Fiber: 3g; Net Carbs: 4g; Protein: 44g; Macros: Fat 56%/Protein 41%/Carbs 3%

Jalapeño-Cheese Hamburger Steaks

Prep time: 10 minutes Cook time: 15 minutes

Simple but so delish, these hamburger steaks are stuffed with onion and jalapeño peppers and are best topped with creamy Ranch Dressing (page 181). Serve with Green Chile Cauliflower "Mac" and Cheese (page 94) or Jalapeño Coleslaw (page 63). **Serves 6**

1½ pounds ground beef

⅓ cup finely diced red onion

1 or 2 jalapeño peppers, seeded and finely diced

1 cup shredded cheddar cheese

3 teaspoons Worcestershire sauce

1 teaspoon garlic powder

1½ teaspoons kosher salt

½ teaspoon freshly ground black pepper

1. In a medium mixing bowl, break apart the ground beef and add the onion, jalapeños, cheddar cheese, Worcestershire sauce, garlic powder, salt, and pepper. Gently combine the ingredients but don't overwork the mixture or the steaks will be dense.

2. Divide the mixture evenly into 6 portions. Use your hands to gently roll each portion into a ball, then flatten into a patty about ¼ inch thick.

3. Preheat a heavy-bottomed skillet over medium-high heat. Cook the patties (three at a time) and sear for about 3 minutes per side, or until they reach your desired doneness. Repeat with the remaining patties.

Tip: Some jalapeños are mild and some are unexpectedly hot, so testing them in advance will help you control the heat level of your dish. Check their heat level when chopping them by tasting a tiny piece. Also, wear disposable gloves while handling peppers to avoid irritation. Wash your hands with cold water and avoid touching your face.

Per Serving Calories: 373; Total Fat: 25g; Total Carbs: 3g; Fiber: <1g; Net Carbs: 3g; Protein: 33g; Macros: Fat 60%/Protein 35%/Carbs 5%

Skillet Beef Potpie

Prep time: 20 minutes Cook time: 50 minutes

This recipe was inspired by my grandma's famous beef pie. This keto version uses sweet, thinly sliced turnips for the crust. **Serves 6**

1½ pounds ground beef

1½ teaspoons kosher salt, divided

1 teaspoon freshly ground black pepper, divided

½ cup diced onion

8 ounces mushrooms, sliced

2 garlic cloves, minced

1 cup beef stock or bone broth

3 tablespoons tomato paste

1 tablespoon Worcestershire sauce

½ teaspoon dried thyme

1½ cups frozen green beans

1 pound turnips, peeled and thinly sliced

1 tablespoon avocado oil or extra-virgin olive oil

1. Preheat the oven to 400°F.

2. In a large oven-safe skillet, heat the ground beef and season with 1 teaspoon salt and ½ teaspoon pepper. Cook over medium-high heat for about 5 minutes. Add the onion, mushrooms, and garlic. Continue to cook until the beef and mushrooms are browned and the onions are tender, 5 to 7 minutes.

3. Stir in the stock, tomato paste, Worcestershire sauce, and thyme and bring to a simmer. Cook for 2 to 3 minutes, then stir in the green beans.

4. Remove from the heat and layer the turnips in a circular pattern on top of the beef mixture. Brush the turnips with the avocado oil and sprinkle with the remaining ½ teaspoon salt and ½ teaspoon pepper.

5. Cover with aluminum foil and bake for 25 minutes. Remove the foil and bake for an additional 10 minutes, or until the turnips are tender and golden. Let stand for 5 minutes before serving.

Per Serving Calories: 367; Total Fat: 21g; Total Carbs: 13g; Fiber: 3g; Net Carbs: 10g; Protein: 32g; Macros: Fat 51%/ Protein 35%/Carbs 14%

Cheeseburger Casserole

Prep time: 10 minutes Cook time: 45 minutes

Cheeseburger Casserole might sound a little strange, but I promise you will not be thinking about the name after one bite. This recipe is one of my go-to choices for family and friends because it is so hearty. You can also whip it up for two people and freeze the leftovers. **Serves 4**

1 pound 80-percent lean ground beef

½ cup diced onion

2 garlic cloves, minced

4 eggs

5 tablespoons tomato paste

½ cup heavy (whipping) cream

½ teaspoon kosher salt

¼ teaspoon freshly ground black pepper

1½ cups shredded cheddar cheese, divided

1. Preheat the oven to 350°F.

2. In a large skillet, brown the ground beef with the onion and garlic for about 10 minutes. Drain the excess grease and spread the beef mixture in the bottom of a 9-inch pie pan or a 9-inch square baking dish.

3. In a medium bowl, whisk together the eggs, tomato paste, heavy cream, salt, and pepper until well combined. Add 1 cup cheddar cheese to the egg mixture and stir to combine. Then pour the mixture over the beef.

4. Top the casserole with the remaining ½ cup cheese and bake for 30 to 35 minutes, or until set and golden brown.

Per Serving Calories: 657; Total Fat: 48g; Total Carbs: 9g; Fiber: 1g; Net Carbs: 8g; Protein: 46g; Macros: Fat 66%/ Protein 28%/Carbs 6%

Beef and Broccoli

Prep time: 10 minutes Cook time: 20 minutes

Skip the takeout and make an upgraded keto version of this popular dish. My friends rave about this recipe, and it will most likely become a keto staple for you. Serve it on its own or with cauliflower rice for an indulgent yet guilt-free meal. **Serves 4**

1 tablespoon coconut oil

1½ pounds skirt steak, cut into 2-inch strips

4 garlic cloves, minced

1½ teaspoons peeled and minced fresh ginger

6 cups broccoli florets

½ cup water

⅓ cup coconut aminos

1 teaspoon rice vinegar

Juice of ½ lemon

Pinch red pepper flakes (optional)

Kosher salt

Freshly ground black pepper

1. In a large skillet, melt the coconut oil over medium-high heat. Sauté the steak for 5 to 7 minutes. Remove from the pan and set aside.

2. Reduce the heat to medium and add the garlic and ginger. Cook and stir until fragrant, about 1 minute. Add the broccoli and cook for 2 minutes, or until lightly browned.

3. Add the water, cover, and reduce the heat to medium-low. Cook for 8 to 10 minutes, stirring occasionally, until the broccoli is tender.

4. Add the coconut aminos, vinegar, lemon juice, red pepper flakes (if using), and the steak to the broccoli. Sauté, tossing to combine, for 1 to 2 minutes. Season with salt and black pepper before serving.

Per Serving Calories: 508; Total Fat: 34g; Total Carbs: 15g; Fiber: 4g; Net Carbs: 11g; Protein: 34g; Macros: Fat 60%/ Protein 27%/Carbs 13%

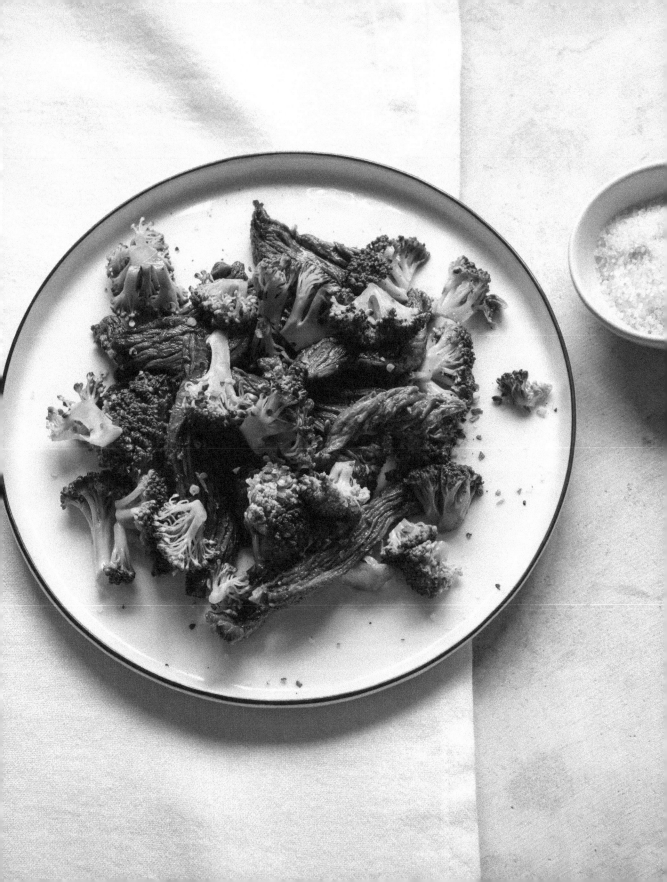

Osso Bucco

Prep time: 10 minutes Cook time: 3 hours 10 minutes

Osso bucco is traditionally prepared with veal, but I prefer using beef shanks for this comfort food classic that's made in just one pot. The beef shanks create their own rich, flavorful sauce that's incredible served over the tender meat, and the whole thing is topped with a classic mixture of fresh parsley, lemon, and garlic. **Serves 4**

3 tablespoons bacon fat or butter

4 crosscut beef shanks

1½ teaspoons kosher salt

1 teaspoon freshly ground black pepper

¾ cup finely chopped onion

1 cup chopped celery

4 garlic cloves, 3 finely chopped and 1 minced

½ cup dry white wine or bone broth

1 cup chopped tomatoes

2 cups beef stock or bone broth

1 bay leaf

½ teaspoon dried basil

½ teaspoon dried thyme

1½ tablespoons chopped fresh parsley

½ teaspoon grated lemon zest

1. Preheat the oven to 325°F.

2. In a Dutch oven or other oven-safe pan, melt the bacon fat over medium-high heat. Season the beef with the salt and pepper, then cook for 3 to 5 minutes on each side, or until browned. Remove the beef and set aside.

3. Add the onion and celery to the pan and cook until the onion is translucent, 4 to 5 minutes. Add the finely chopped garlic and cook for another minute. Deglaze the pot with the wine, scraping up any browned bits from the bottom, and cook until the liquid is reduced by half.

4. Add the tomatoes, stock, bay leaf, basil, and thyme and return the beef to the pot. Cover and place on the center rack of the oven. Bake for 2½ to 3 hours, or until the beef is tender.

5. Meanwhile, in a small bowl, combine the parsley, lemon zest, and minced garlic. Set aside

6. When the beef is done cooking, remove it from the pot and place on a serving platter. Discard the bay leaf. Using an immersion blender, puree the vegetables and remaining stock. Pour the sauce over the beef and sprinkle the parsley mixture over top.

Per Serving Calories: 290; Total Fat: 14g; Total Carbs: 7g; Fiber: 2g; Net Carbs: 5g; Protein: 27g; Macros: Fat 43%/ Protein 37%/Carbs 20%

New Orleans Dirty Rice

Prep time: 10 minutes Cook time: 20 minutes

Bring a little taste of Louisiana to your dinner table with this quick and easy cauliflower rice dish. Full of Cajun flavors, this is a skillet meal that will have your family, keto or not, begging for more. **Serves 4**

3 tablespoons bacon fat

1½ pounds ground beef

1½ teaspoons kosher salt, divided

¼ teaspoon freshly ground black pepper

1 teaspoon garlic powder, divided

1 cup diced celery

½ cup diced bell pepper

½ cup diced onion

3 garlic cloves, finely minced

¾ teaspoon paprika

¼ teaspoon dried oregano

¼ teaspoon dried thyme

¼ teaspoon cayenne pepper

1 (12-ounce) bag frozen cauliflower rice

¼ cup chicken stock

3 scallions, both white and green parts, sliced

1. In a large, heavy-bottomed skillet, melt the bacon fat over medium-high heat. Add the ground beef and season with 1 teaspoon salt, the black pepper, and ½ teaspoon garlic powder. Cook the beef for 8 to 10 minutes, breaking it apart with a spoon, until it begins to brown and caramelize.

2. Reduce the heat to medium and add the celery, bell pepper, and onion and continue to cook for about 5 minutes, or until the vegetables are tender and the onions are translucent. Add the garlic, paprika, oregano, thyme, and cayenne pepper and cook for another minute.

3. Add the cauliflower rice and stock and season with the remaining ½ teaspoon salt and ½ teaspoon garlic powder. Stir to combine, using the stock and the liquid from the cauliflower to deglaze the pan, scraping up any browned bits from the bottom.

4. Continue to cook, stirring often, until the cauliflower rice is tender and there is no liquid left in the pan, 4 to 5 minutes. Taste and adjust the seasoning as needed. Sprinkle with scallions and serve.

Tip: Pork breakfast sausage works perfectly in this dish in place of ground beef, and it's a great way to use any surplus you may have in the freezer.

Per Serving Calories: 569; Total Fat: 37g; Total Carbs: 11g; Fiber: 4g; Net Carbs: 7g; Protein: 46g; Macros: Fat 58%/Protein 32%/Carbs 10%

Sweet Italian Sausage with Caramelized Cabbage

Prep time: 5 minutes Cook time: 30 minutes

Sausage and cabbage are an ideal culinary match for a simple but delicious family-friendly keto dinner. Look for fresh Italian sausage at the butcher's counter. Be sure to keep the skillet cooking over low heat, which will ensure the sausage is browned and the cabbage is caramelized and sweet. **Serves 4**

2 tablespoons bacon fat or avocado oil

4 fresh sweet Italian sausages

6 cups finely sliced green cabbage

1½ teaspoons kosher salt, divided

1 teaspoon granulated garlic, divided

½ teaspoon freshly ground black pepper, divided

3 scallions, both white and light green parts, sliced

1. In a large skillet, melt the bacon fat over medium-low heat. Add the sausages and cover them with 3 cups sliced cabbage. Season the cabbage with 1 teaspoon salt, ½ teaspoon garlic, and ¼ teaspoon pepper, stirring the cabbage on occasion to make sure it doesn't burn. Add the remaining 3 cups cabbage and season with the remaining ½ teaspoon salt, ½ teaspoon garlic, and ¼ teaspoon pepper.

2. Cover and cook over low to medium-low heat for about 20 minutes. Remove the lid and continue to cook, stirring often, for another 5 to 10 minutes, or until the sausage is browned on all sides and the cabbage is tender and begins to brown and caramelize. Top with the scallions and serve.

Tip: This recipe would also be fantastic with bulk Italian sausage, if you can't find it in the casing. Simply cook the sausage meat until browned, add the cabbage and seasonings, stirring the cabbage on occasion to make sure it doesn't burn, and continue to step 2.

Per Serving Calories: 223; Total Fat: 14g; Total Carbs: 11g; Fiber: 3g; Net Carbs: 8g; Protein: 16g; Macros: Fat 56%/ Protein 29%/Carbs 15%

Pork Belly Burnt Ends

Prep time: 10 minutes Cook time: 4 hours

Burnt ends are smoky, sweet, and sticky, super tender bites of beef brisket that are a barbecue delicacy in Texas. This low-carb meaty version is made with flavorful pork belly, which should be easy to find in your local grocery store's meat department. Slow smoked and simmered in sugar-free barbecue sauce, these decadent bites of pork are perfect served with Classic Fauxtato Salad (page 61) or Jalapeño Coleslaw (page 63). **Serves 8**

3 pounds pork belly

1 teaspoon granulated garlic

½ teaspoon onion powder

3 teaspoons kosher salt

2 teaspoons freshly ground black pepper

2 teaspoons paprika

1 cup sugar-free barbecue sauce

⅓ cup water

1. Preheat a smoker, grill, or oven to 225°F. If you're cooking in the oven, line a baking sheet with aluminum foil and place a metal baking rack on top.

2. Trim the skin and the top layer of fat off the pork belly. In a small bowl, combine the garlic, onion powder, salt, pepper, and paprika and season the pork belly all over with the mixture. Place the seasoned belly on the smoker or grill rack and cover. If you're cooking in the oven, place the pork belly on the rack in the baking sheet. Cook for 2 to 3 hours, or until the internal temperature of the pork reaches 190°F to 195°F.

3. Remove the pork belly from the smoker, grill, or oven and cut into 2-inch cubes. Place the cubes in a disposable aluminum pan or, if you're using the oven, a 3-quart casserole dish. In a small bowl, combine the barbecue sauce and water and pour it over the pork cubes.

continued >

4. Cover the pan with foil and return it to the smoker, grill, or oven. Cook for 45 minutes, then remove the foil and cook for another 10 to 15 minutes, or until the sauce is thickened and the pork has reached an internal temperature of 200°F to 205°F.

Tip: Barbecue sauce is what glazes these burnt ends and creates a delicious sticky coating. Use a sugar-free sauce that still has some sweetness, as opposed to a vinegar-based sauce.

Per Serving Calories: 896; Total Fat: 90g; Total Carbs: 5g; Fiber: <1g; Net Carbs: 5g; Protein: 16g; Macros: Fat 90%/Protein 7%/Carbs 3%

Chipotle-Lime Pork Tenderloin

Prep time: 5 minutes Cook time: 25 minutes

Pork tenderloins are inexpensive and cook fast, which makes them great for a quick keto dinner. Bold and spicy, these pork tenderloins are packed with chipotle, garlic, and lime flavors. Pair with Sautéed Summer Squash (page 86) for a meal that will spice up your weeknight. **Serves 6**

4 garlic cloves, finely minced

2 canned chipotle peppers in adobo sauce, finely chopped, plus 3 tablespoons adobo sauce

1 teaspoon grated lime zest

½ cup freshly squeezed lime juice

2 teaspoons granulated 1:1 sweetener

2 (1- to 1½-pound) pork tenderloins

1½ teaspoons kosher salt

1 teaspoon chili powder

½ teaspoon ground cumin

1 teaspoon garlic powder

2 tablespoons avocado oil

1. Preheat the oven to 400°F.

2. In a small bowl, combine the garlic, chipotle peppers, adobo sauce, lime zest, lime juice, and sweetener and mix well to combine. Set aside

3. Rub the pork tenderloin all over with the salt, chili powder, cumin, and garlic powder. Preheat a large oven-safe skillet over medium-high heat. Pour in the avocado oil and sear the pork for 2 to 3 minutes per side, or until brown.

4. Brush the pork with the chipotle glaze and put the skillet in the oven. Roast for 15 minutes, or until the internal temperature reaches at least 145°F, generously brushing with the glaze every 5 minutes while roasting. Remove from the oven, cover loosely with aluminum foil, and let the pork rest for at least 5 minutes before slicing.

Tip: Pork tenderloin is also great on the grill. Preheat the grill to 400°F and season the pork as described. Place the seasoned pork on the hot grill and baste often with the glaze while grilling. Cook until the meat reaches the desired doneness, 15 to 20 minutes, then remove from the grill, cover loosely with foil, and let the pork rest for 5 to 10 minutes before slicing.

Per Serving Calories: 230; Total Fat: 7g; Total Carbs: 7g; Fiber: 1g; Net Carbs: 5g; Protein: 34g; Macros: Fat 27%/ Protein 59%/Carbs 14%

Pot Sticker Meatballs

Prep time: 10 minutes Cook time: 20 minutes

When I'm craving my favorite pot stickers, I whip up a batch of these flavor-packed meatballs instead. Loaded with garlic, ginger, and scallions and served with a spicy dipping sauce, these meatballs have all the flavor of pot stickers without the wrapper. They're perfect for serving to a crowd as an appetizer or as a meal along with Fried Cauliflower Rice (page 92). This recipe makes 30 meatballs. **Serves 6**

1½ pounds ground pork

1 cup finely chopped Napa cabbage

3 garlic cloves, grated

2 scallions, both white and green parts, finely chopped

3 teaspoons sesame oil, divided

1½ tablespoons grated fresh ginger

2 tablespoons plus ½ cup soy sauce or liquid aminos

1 egg, beaten

2 tablespoons coconut flour

2 teaspoons sriracha

2½ tablespoons rice wine vinegar or apple cider vinegar

1 teaspoon granulated 1:1 sweetener

1. Preheat the oven to 450°F. Line a large baking sheet with parchment paper.

2. In a large bowl, combine the pork, cabbage, garlic, scallions, 2 teaspoons sesame oil, ginger, 2 tablespoons soy sauce, egg, and coconut flour. Mix well to combine.

3. Using a cookie scoop, form the pork mixture into golf ball–size meatballs and place them on the prepared baking sheet. Repeat until all the pork mixture is used. Bake for 15 to 18 minutes, or until the meatballs are browned.

4. Meanwhile, in a small bowl, mix together the remaining 1 teaspoon sesame oil, sriracha, remaining ½ cup soy sauce, vinegar, and sweetener. Serve the meatballs warm with the dipping sauce.

Per Serving Calories: 365; Total Fat: 28g; Total Carbs: 6g; Fiber: 1g; Net Carbs: 5g; Protein: 23g; Macros: Fat 69%/ Protein 25%/Carbs 6%30 Minutes or Less, Dairy-Free

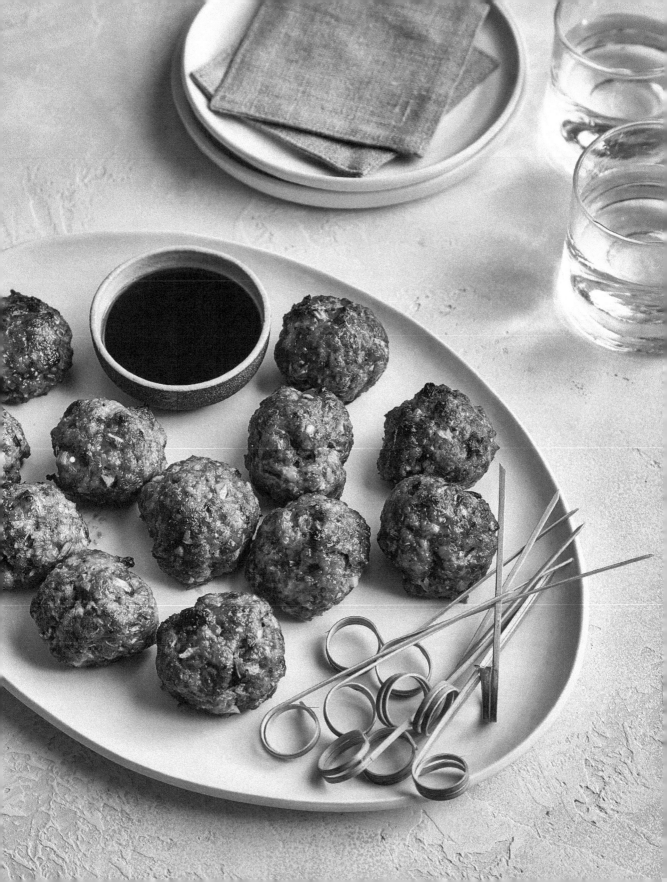

German-Style Ham Rolls

Prep time: 10 minutes Cook time: 20 minutes

No bread needed for this Reuben-inspired dish, which offers the flavors of the classic ham and cheese sandwich with a fraction of the carbs. **Serves 4**

3 tablespoons butter, plus more for greasing

¼ cup diced onion

2 cups German-style sauerkraut, drained

¼ teaspoon kosher salt, plus a pinch

¼ teaspoon freshly ground black pepper

8 deli ham slices

2½ tablespoons whole-grain mustard

1½ cups shredded Gruyère, baby Swiss, or Havarti cheese

½ cup keto-friendly mayonnaise or Three-Minute Mayo (page 178)

2 tablespoons sugar-free sweet pickle relish

2 tablespoons sugar-free ketchup

¼ teaspoon onion powder

1 teaspoon Worcestershire sauce

1. Preheat the oven to 400°F. Lightly grease a 9-by-13-inch baking dish with butter.

2. In a medium skillet, melt the butter over medium heat. Add the onion and sauté for 3 to 4 minutes, or until translucent. Add the sauerkraut and season with ¼ teaspoon salt and the pepper. Cook until no liquid remains, about 5 minutes.

3. Smear each slice of ham with about 1 teaspoon mustard and top with ¼ cup of the sauerkraut mixture. Sprinkle with 2 tablespoons shredded cheese. Roll the ham up, jelly roll–style, and place seam-side down in the prepared baking dish. Repeat with the remaining ham slices. Top with the remaining cheese.

4. Bake for 10 to 12 minutes, until the cheese is melted.

5. In a small bowl, stir together the mayonnaise, relish, ketchup, onion powder, Worcestershire sauce, and a pinch salt. Serve the rolls warm, topped with the sauce.

Per Serving Calories: 558; Total Fat: 46g; Total Carbs: 14g; Fiber: 4g; Net Carbs: 10g; Protein: 23g; Macros: Fat 74%/Protein 16%/Carbs 10%

Creamy Parmesan Pork Chops

Prep time: 5 minutes Cook time: 25 minutes

A fabulous way to add some flavor to pork chops is with a creamy Parmesan sauce. Like red meat, pork is rich in protein and fat and contains many nutrients, including vitamin B$_{12}$, potassium, iron, magnesium, and zinc. This recipe pairs well with Pan-Roasted Red Radish "Potatoes" (page 98). **Serves 6**

2 tablespoons extra-virgin olive oil

6 (5-ounce) center-cut boneless pork chops

½ onion, sliced

2 garlic cloves, minced

1 cup heavy (whipping) cream

½ cup shredded mozzarella cheese

⅓ cup chicken stock

⅓ cup grated Parmesan cheese

2 tablespoons cream cheese, at room temperature

1 tablespoon Italian seasoning

½ teaspoon kosher salt

½ teaspoon freshly ground black pepper

1. In a large skillet, heat the olive oil over medium-high heat. Add the pork chops, onion, and garlic. Cook the pork chops for about 4 minutes per side.

2. Remove the pork chops from the skillet and add the heavy cream, mozzarella cheese, stock, Parmesan cheese, cream cheese, Italian seasoning, salt, and pepper. Reduce the heat to medium and cook until the sauce thickens, stirring constantly, for about 8 minutes.

3. Return the pork chops to the sauce, reduce the heat to low, and simmer for about 5 minutes to heat through.

Tip: Make sure the cream cheese is softened to prevent lumps in the sauce.

Per Serving Calories: 467; Total Fat: 36g; Total Carbs: 6g; Fiber: <1g; Net Carbs: 6g; Protein: 32g; Macros: Fat 69%/ Protein 27%/Carbs 4%

Egg Roll in a Bowl

Prep time: 5 minutes Cook time: 15 minutes

This quick dish gives you all the flavors of an egg roll without the fried non-keto wrapper. You can use a fresh head of cabbage and slice it thin, but for convenience you can also pick up a couple bags of coleslaw mix. It contains a few slivers of carrots, but not enough to throw off the carb count of the final dish. The sesame oil has a rich, smoky flavor and really adds to the Asian-inspired flavor profile, but it's not absolutely necessary. If you happen to have some or want to try it, be sure to add it at the end of cooking and toss well to combine. **Serves 6**

2 tablespoons extra-virgin olive oil

2 pounds ground pork

½ small onion, sliced thinly

3 garlic cloves, minced

½ teaspoon kosher salt

½ teaspoon freshly ground black pepper

6 cups shredded cabbage or coleslaw mix

3 or 4 dashes hot sauce

2 teaspoons granulated 1:1 sweetener

2 tablespoons coconut aminos or soy sauce

2 teaspoons sesame oil (optional)

1. In a large skillet, heat the olive oil over medium-high heat. Add the pork, onion, garlic, salt, and pepper. Cook until the meat is browned, about 10 minutes.

2. Add the coleslaw mix and toss with the meat. Add the hot sauce, sweetener, and coconut aminos and toss well to coat. Sauté over medium-high heat for 5 to 7 minutes, or until the cabbage is wilted and the dish is well combined.

3. Remove from the heat and drizzle the sesame oil (if using) over the dish. Toss to combine and serve warm.

Tip: Ground pork is great for this dish, but any ground or minced meat will work, including beef, turkey, and chicken.

Per Serving Calories: 460; Total Fat: 37g; Total Carbs: 7g; Fiber: 2g; Net Carbs: 3g; Protein: 26g; Macros: Fat 72%/ Protein 23%/Carbs 5%

Herbed Lamb Chops

Prep time: 5 minutes Cook time: 15 minutes

Fresh herbs and garlic infuse these succulent lamb chops with amazing flavor. Look for loin chops, which are more tender than sirloin chops. Serve these herbed chops with Loaded Cauliflower Mash (page 97) or Pan-Roasted Red Radish "Potatoes" (page 98). **Serves 4**

8 lamb loin chops, about 1 inch thick

2 teaspoons kosher salt

1 teaspoon freshly ground black pepper

¼ cup finely chopped fresh parsley

1½ tablespoons chopped fresh rosemary

3 scallions, both white and green parts, finely chopped

2 tablespoons avocado oil or extra-virgin olive oil

3 garlic cloves, minced

3 tablespoons butter

1. If desired, trim any excess fat from the lamb chops. Let them come to room temperature. Season both sides with the salt and pepper. In a small bowl, combine the parsley, rosemary, and scallions and rub the mixture onto both sides of the chops.

2. In a large skillet, heat the avocado oil over medium-high heat until it shimmers. Add the lamb chops and cook for 2 to 3 minutes on each side, or until browned.

3. Reduce the heat to medium-low and add the garlic and butter to the pan. Spoon the butter and garlic over the lamp chops and continue to cook for 4 to 5 minutes, or until the internal temperature reaches 125°F for medium-rare or to your desired doneness.

4. Remove the chops from the pan, loosely cover with aluminum foil, and let rest for at least 5 minutes before serving.

Per Serving Calories: 787; Total Fat: 68g; Total Carbs: 2g; Fiber: 1g; Net Carbs: 1g; Protein: 39g; Macros: Fat 78%/ Protein 20%/Carbs 2%

Greek-Style Lamb Burgers

Prep time: 20 minutes Cook time: 10 minutes

Shake things up on burger night with these juicy, flavorful Greek-inspired lamb burgers, seasoned with aromatic herbs and spices. Serve these burgers wrapped in romaine lettuce topped with sliced tomato and cucumbers, feta cheese, and creamy tzatziki sauce, with Eggplant Fries (page 91) on the side. **Serves 6**

FOR THE TZATZIKI SAUCE

¼ cup grated English cucumber

1 garlic clove, finely minced or grated

1 teaspoon freshly squeezed lemon juice

½ teaspoon grated lemon zest

¾ cup plain full-fat Greek yogurt

1 teaspoon extra-virgin olive oil

¼ teaspoon kosher salt

¼ teaspoon freshly ground black pepper

FOR THE BURGERS

2 pounds ground lamb

¼ cup grated red onion

2 garlic cloves, finely minced

½ cup chopped fresh parsley

TO MAKE THE TZATZIKI SAUCE

1. In a small bowl, combine the cucumber, garlic, lemon juice, lemon zest, yogurt, olive oil, salt, and pepper and stir to combine. Cover and refrigerate.

TO MAKE THE BURGERS

2. Preheat the grill to 400°F to 425°F.

3. In a large mixing bowl, combine the lamb, onion, garlic, parsley, mint, oregano, cumin, paprika, salt, pepper, and olive oil and mix thoroughly, making sure not to overmix. Using your hands, divide the mixture into 6 portions and form into patties about ¼ to ½ inch thick.

4. Grill the burgers for 4 to 6 minutes per side, or until the internal temperature reaches 160°F for medium or to the desired doneness. Or heat a large skillet over medium-high heat and sear the burgers for 3 to 5 minutes per side.

3 tablespoons chopped
fresh mint

1½ teaspoons dried oregano

2 teaspoons ground cumin

1 teaspoon paprika

1½ teaspoons kosher salt

¾ teaspoon freshly ground
black pepper

1 tablespoon extra-virgin
olive oil

5. Let the patties rest for at least 5 minutes. Serve topped with tzatziki sauce.

Tip: For deliciously tender burgers, don't press on the burgers while cooking and flip only once while cooking.

Per Serving Calories: 493; Total Fat: 40g; Total Carbs: 4g; Fiber: 1g; Net Carbs: 3g; Protein: 28g; Macros: Fat 73%/Protein 23%/Carbs 4%

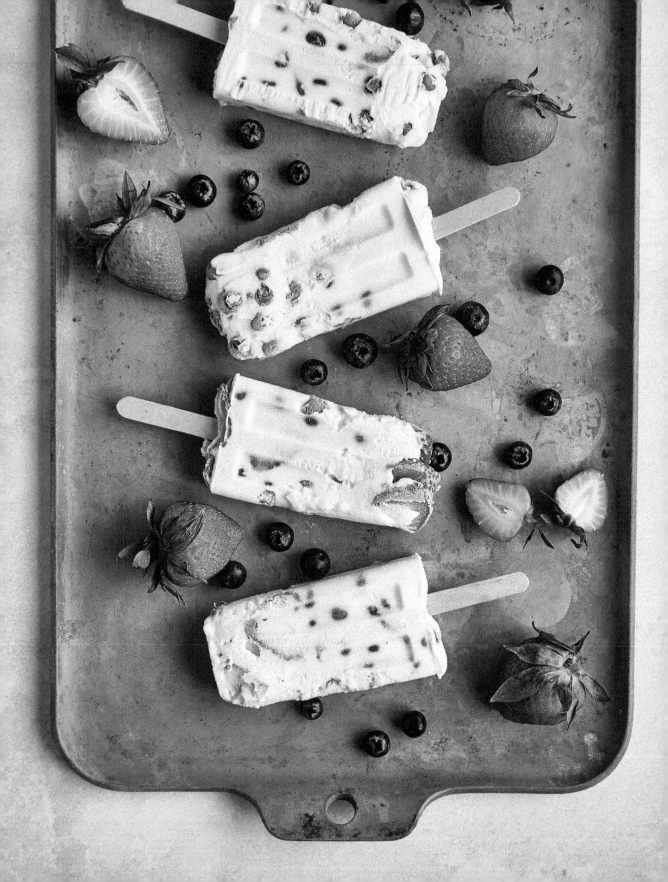

Desserts

Strawberries and Cream Ice Pops, page 170

Butter Pecan Mousse

Prep time: 15 minutes, plus 2 hours to chill Cook time: 5 minutes

If you're a fan of butter pecan ice cream, you're going to fall in love with this delicious dessert. Roasted pecans, vanilla, and caramelized browned butter shine in this quick and easy mousse. Make a batch and keep in it in the refrigerator for when you crave something sweet. **Serves 4**

1½ tablespoons butter

¼ cup pecans, finely chopped

4 ounces cream cheese, at room temperature

3 tablespoons powdered 1:1 sweetener

1 teaspoon vanilla extract

½ cup heavy (whipping) cream

1. In a small skillet, combine the butter and pecans and cook over medium-low heat until the pecans are toasted and the butter is browned, 5 to 6 minutes. Remove from the heat. Transfer the pecans and any browned bits from the skillet to a small bowl and set aside.

2. Using a handheld mixer in a medium bowl, combine the cream cheese, sweetener, and vanilla and beat until light and fluffy. Stir in the cooled pecans and set aside.

3. In another bowl, whip the heavy cream until soft peaks form. Gently fold the whipped cream into the cream cheese mixture. Spoon into four serving dishes and refrigerate for at least 2 hours before serving.

Per Serving Calories: 286; Total Fat: 30g; Total Carbs: 15g; Fiber: 1g; Net Carbs: 3g; Protein: 3g; Macros: Fat 94%/ Protein 4%/Carbs 2%

Macerated Berries with Lime and Coconut Cream

Prep time: 10 minutes, plus 30 minutes to macerate

This simple no-cook dessert is a great option for warmer weather or when you want something light and refreshing. Prepare the berries in advance so they are ready and waiting to be dished up. Use any combination of fresh berries you like, but limit blueberries as they are higher in carbs. Garnish with a little extra lime zest, if you'd like. **Serves 6**

1 cup raspberries

1 cup blackberries

1 cup strawberries, halved or quartered

3 to 5 tablespoons powdered 1:1 sweetener, divided

Grated zest of ½ lime

2 teaspoons freshly squeezed lime juice

1 cup coconut cream

¼ teaspoon vanilla extract

1. In a medium bowl, mix the raspberries, blackberries, and strawberries and toss with 1 to 2 tablespoons sweetener, the lime zest, and lime juice. Let sit for at least 30 minutes.

2. In a medium bowl, whip the coconut cream until light and fluffy. Add 2 to 3 tablespoons sweetener (more or less, depending on how sweet you like it) and the vanilla and whip for another minute.

3. Serve the berries topped with the coconut cream.

Tip: Canned coconut cream is widely available in most grocery stores. This is different than cream of coconut, which is very sweet. Do not shake the can before opening it, and spoon out only the solid coconut cream from the top, leaving the clear liquid in the can. Including the clear liquid will prevent the cream from whipping up. Refrigerate the liquid to use in smoothies.

Per Serving Calories: 97; Total Fat: 7g; Total Carbs: 16g; Fiber: 3g; Net Carbs: 5g; Protein: 1g; Macros: Fat 65%/ Protein 4%/Carbs 31%

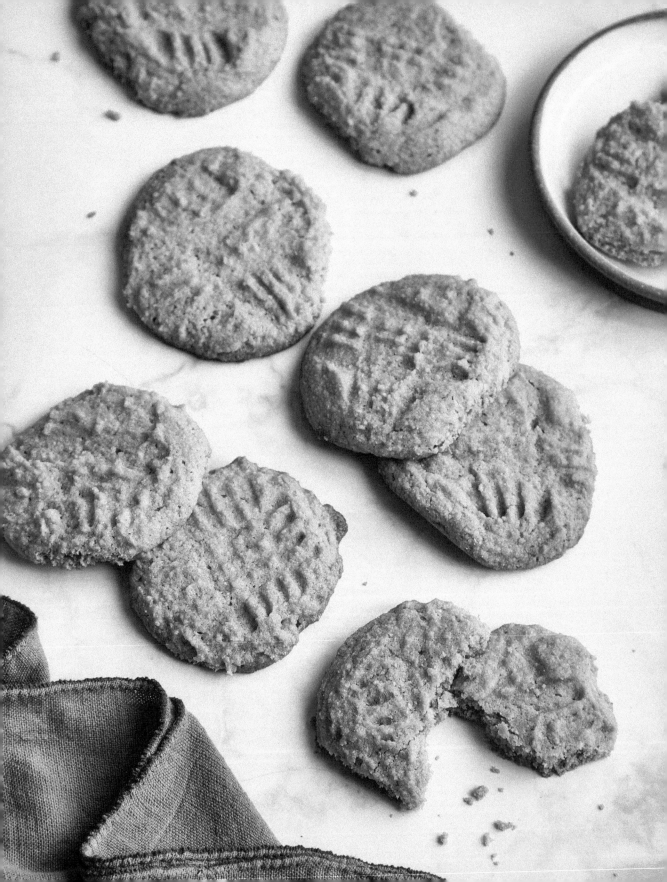

Ultimate Peanut Butter Cookies

Prep time: 10 minutes, plus 15 minutes to chill Cook time: 8 minutes

If you love peanut butter cookies like I do, stop everything and get out your mixing bowl. I don't use the word "ultimate" lightly. These are soft, chewy, and crisp on the edges, with amazing peanut butter flavor—everything you expect in the ultimate cookie! **Makes about 24 cookies**

1 cup almond flour

2 tablespoons coconut flour

¼ teaspoon kosher salt

¾ teaspoon baking soda

1 tablespoon unflavored powdered gelatin

8 tablespoons (1 stick) butter, at room temperature

⅔ cup creamy no-sugar-added peanut butter, at room temperature

½ cup granulated 1:1 sweetener

1 egg, at room temperature

½ teaspoon vanilla extract

1. Preheat the oven to 350°F. Line a large baking sheet with parchment paper.

2. In a medium bowl, mix together the almond flour, coconut flour, salt, baking soda, and gelatin. Set aside.

3. Using a handheld mixer in a large bowl, combine the butter, peanut butter, and sweetener and beat until well combined. Add the egg and vanilla and mix well. Add the almond flour mixture and stir until thoroughly combined. Refrigerate the dough for 10 to 15 minutes.

4. Scoop about 1½ tablespoons of dough at a time onto the prepared baking sheet, pressing down lightly with a fork or your hand to flatten it into a cookie.

5. Bake for 8 minutes. Cool the cookies completely on the baking sheet. Store in a covered container at room temperature for up to 4 days.

Tip: If you're a chocolate lover, stir ½ cup of sugar-free semisweet chocolate chips into the dough before chilling.

Per Serving (1 cookie) Calories: 110; Total Fat: 10g; Total Carbs: 7g; Fiber: 1g; Net Carbs: 2g; Protein: 3g; Macros: Fat 82%/Protein 11%/Carbs 7%

Coconut Crème Brûlée

Prep time: 10 minutes Cook time: 35 minutes

Crème brûlée is one of my all-time favorite desserts, and this keto version is just as delicious as the traditional recipe but has no sugar or dairy. Using coconut milk instead of cream lends incredible flavor to this decadent treat. Keto-friendly sugar alternatives don't caramelize very well, so this version is topped with toasted coconut for a little crunch. **Serves 6**

1 (13.5-ounce) can full-fat coconut milk

6 tablespoons granulated 1:1 sweetener

Pinch kosher salt

1½ teaspoons vanilla extract

6 egg yolks

⅓ cup toasted unsweetened coconut

1. Preheat the oven to 375°F.

2. In a saucepan, combine the coconut milk, sweetener, and salt over medium heat. Cook until the sweetener is dissolved and the milk is almost at a simmer. Remove from the heat, stir in the vanilla, and set aside.

3. Meanwhile, using a stand mixer or handheld mixer in a large bowl, beat the egg yolks until thickened and light in color, about 2 minutes. With the mixer on low, slowly add the coconut milk mixture to the egg yolks.

4. Place 6 ramekins in a 9-by-13-inch baking pan and evenly pour the custard into the ramekins. Place the pan in the oven and add boiling water to the pan to a depth of 1 inch.

5. Bake for 25 to 30 minutes, or until the custard is set. Remove the ramekins from the water and cool on a wire rack. Cover and chill until you're ready to serve. Just before serving, divide the toasted coconut evenly over the tops of the custards.

Tip: Do not skip the water bath when baking the custard. The water helps insulate the ramekins while baking, which ensures a creamy, velvety custard.

Per Serving Calories: 192; Total Fat: 19g; Total Carbs: 15g; Fiber: 1g; Net Carbs: 2g; Protein: 3g; Macros: Fat 89%/ Protein 6%/Carbs 5%

Grasshopper Fudge Fat Bombs

Prep time: 10 minutes, plus 1 hour to chill Cook time: 5 minutes

Fat bombs are great to have on hand in the refrigerator or freezer for when cravings hit. These minty, fudgy bites taste just like those cookies you know and love and will most definitely satisfy your sweet cravings. I enjoy them straight from the freezer. **Makes 32 fat bombs**

5 ounces sugar-free dark or semisweet chocolate chips

Pinch kosher salt

¼ teaspoon peppermint extract

⅓ cup coconut oil

⅓ cup granulated 1:1 allulose blend sweetener

½ cup heavy (whipping) cream

1. Line an 8- or 9-inch loaf pan with plastic wrap and set aside. In a medium bowl, combine the chocolate chips, salt, and peppermint extract and set aside.

2. In a saucepan, combine the coconut oil and sweetener over medium heat. Bring to a rolling boil and cook for about 1 minute. Add the heavy cream, return to a boil, and cook for an additional minute. Set aside to cool for 5 minutes.

3. Pour the warm coconut oil mixture over the chocolate chips. Let sit for 1 minute, then stir until smooth and the chocolate is completely melted.

4. Pour immediately into the prepared loaf pan, spread evenly, and refrigerate until firm, 45 minutes to 1 hour. Cut into 32 pieces.

Per Serving (1 fat bomb) Calories: 48; Total Fat: 5g; Total Carbs: 5g; Fiber: 1g; Net Carbs: 2g; Protein: <1g; Macros: Fat 94%/Protein 0%/Carbs 6%

Gooey Mocha Fudge Cakes

Prep time: 5 minutes Cook time: 15 minutes

If you're obsessed with chocolate like I am, you're going to keep coming back to these coffee-laced individual fudge cakes. The secret to getting a gooey center is to bake the cake until it's puffed and the outside edges are set but the center still has some jiggle. Serve topped with whipped coconut cream or keto vanilla ice cream. **Serves 4**

2 tablespoons butter, melted, plus more for greasing

¼ cup almond flour

1 teaspoon baking powder

¼ cup unsweetened cocoa powder

1½ teaspoons instant espresso

7 tablespoons powdered 1:1 sweetener

⅛ teaspoon kosher salt

2 eggs

½ cup heavy (whipping) cream

2 teaspoons vanilla extract

1. Preheat the oven to 350°F. Lightly grease four 8-ounce ramekins with butter.

2. In a medium bowl, whisk together the almond flour, baking powder, cocoa powder, espresso, sweetener, and salt. Add the eggs, heavy cream, vanilla, and butter and whisk until the batter is smooth and well combined. Divide the batter between the prepared ramekins.

3. Bake for 10 to 13 minutes, or until the edges appear firm and the center is still jiggly. Let the cakes sit for at least 5 minutes before serving.

Tip: These fudge cakes can also be cooked quickly in the microwave. Cook each cake on high for 45 seconds to 1 minute, depending on the wattage of your microwave.

Per Serving Calories: 240; Total Fat: 23g; Total Carbs: 32g; Fiber: 3g; Net Carbs: 3g; Protein: 6g; Macros: Fat 86%/ Protein 10%/Carbs 4%

Pumpkin Spice Cupcakes

Prep time: 10 minutes Cook time: 20 minutes

Easy to make and super moist, these cupcakes are packed with warm, comforting spices and pumpkin flavor. As if that weren't enough, they're topped with a tangy, fluffy keto cream cheese frosting. You'll be making these cupcakes on repeat. **Makes 9 cupcakes**

4 eggs

½ cup almond flour

⅓ cup coconut flour

¼ teaspoon kosher salt

½ cup plain pumpkin puree

1 teaspoon baking powder

½ teaspoon baking soda

¼ cup granulated
1:1 sweetener

½ teaspoon ground
cinnamon

½ teaspoon pumpkin
pie spice

1½ teaspoons vanilla
extract, divided

2 tablespoons sour cream

5 tablespoons butter,
3 melted and 2 at room
temperature

4 ounces cream cheese, at
room temperature

5 tablespoons powdered
1:1 sweetener

1 tablespoon heavy
(whipping) cream

1. Preheat the oven to 350°F. Line a standard muffin pan with 9 cupcake liners.

2. Using a stand mixer with the whisk attachment or a handheld mixer and a large bowl, whip the eggs until light and foamy, about 2 minutes.

3. Add the almond flour, coconut flour, salt, pumpkin, baking powder, baking soda, granulated sweetener, cinnamon, pumpkin pie spice, and 1 teaspoon vanilla and mix on medium speed until everything is combined, scraping down the sides at least once. Stir the sour cream and melted butter into the batter and mix until thoroughly combined.

4. Divide the batter evenly among the lined cups. Bake for 20 to 22 minutes, or until a toothpick inserted in the center of a cupcake comes out clean. Cool the cupcakes in the pan for 5 minutes, then place on a rack to cool completely.

5. Meanwhile, prepare the frosting. Using a stand mixer or a handheld mixer in a medium bowl, cream the cream cheese and room-temperature butter until combined. Add the powdered sweetener and remaining ½ teaspoon vanilla and continue to beat on low speed until the sweetener is well combined. Add the heavy cream and beat on high until it becomes fluffy, 1 to 2 minutes.

6. When the cupcakes are cool, spread about 1½ tablespoons cream cheese frosting on the top of each cupcake.

Tip: Store these cupcakes in a covered container in the refrigerator for up to 4 days or on the counter overnight.

Per Serving (1 cupcake) Calories: 203; Total Fat: 18g; Total Carbs: 20g; Fiber: 3g; Net Carbs: 3g; Protein: 5g; Macros: Fat 80%/Protein 10%/Carbs 10%

Keto Muddy Buddies

Prep time: 10 minutes, plus 30 minutes to chill Cook time: 30 seconds

You may call them by a different name: puppy chow, reindeer chow, monkey munch, or muddy munch. But you know exactly what yummy, sweet snack I'm talking about. With pork rinds in place of the rice cereal, these crunchy morsels are coated with peanut butter and chocolate and then tossed in powdered sweetener. They're so easy to make and will be a favorite snack of kids and adults alike. **Makes 2 cups**

2 cups pork rinds, broken into bite-size pieces

2 ounces sugar-free semisweet chocolate chips

2 tablespoons creamy no-sugar-added peanut butter

1 tablespoon butter

½ teaspoon vanilla extract

7 to 9 tablespoons powdered 1:1 sweetener

1. Place the pork rind pieces in a medium bowl.

2. In a small bowl, combine the chocolate chips, peanut butter, and butter and microwave for 30 seconds, or until everything is melted and smooth. Stir in the vanilla and mix well.

3. Pour the chocolate mixture over the pork rinds and toss to evenly coat.

4. Transfer the coated pork rinds to a large zip-top bag, add the powdered sweetener, seal the bag, and shake until the pieces are well coated.

5. Pour the coated pork rinds onto a small baking sheet and refrigerate for at least 30 minutes to cool and set.

Tip: A confectioners'-style powdered sweetener will give these classic treats their distinctive "powdered" look. Depending on the brand of sweetener you use, you may need to use a few additional tablespoons to coat the pork rinds well.

Per Serving (½ cup) Calories: 212; Total Fat: 16g; Total Carbs: 22g; Fiber: 2g; Net Carbs: 9g; Protein: 12g; Macros: Fat 68%/Protein 23%/Carbs 9%

Snickerdoodle Bars

Prep time: 10 minutes Cook time: 35 minutes

These snickerdoodle bars are buttery and soft with the perfect amount of tang, which is the sign of a good snickerdoodle. Store any leftovers in the refrigerator for up to 5 days or in the freezer for up to 3 weeks.

Makes 24 bars

8 tablespoons (1 stick) unsalted butter, at room temperature, plus more for greasing

2 cups plus 3 tablespoons granulated 1:1 sweetener

8 ounces cream cheese, at room temperature

2 teaspoons vanilla extract

5 eggs, at room temperature

1 cup almond flour, measured and sifted

⅓ cup coconut flour

½ teaspoon baking soda

½ teaspoon cream of tartar

¼ teaspoon kosher salt

2 teaspoons ground cinnamon

1. Preheat the oven to 350°F. Grease a 10-inch square baking pan with butter.

2. Using a handheld mixer on medium speed in a large bowl, beat together 2 cups sweetener, the cream cheese, butter, and vanilla. Add the eggs, one at a time, mixing well after each addition. Fold in the almond flour, coconut flour, baking soda, cream of tartar, and salt.

3. Pour the batter into the prepared pan and spread evenly.

4. In a small bowl, combine the remaining 3 tablespoons sweetener and the cinnamon. Sprinkle the mixture on top of the batter. Bake for 30 to 35 minutes, or until golden brown.

5. Let cool completely in the pan on a wire rack before cutting into bars.

Per Serving (1 bar) Calories: 115; Total Fat: 11g; Total Carbs: 20g; Fiber: 1g; Net Carbs: 2g; Protein: 3g; Macros: Fat 86%/Protein 10%/Carbs 4%

Strawberries and Cream Ice Pops

Prep time: 10 minutes, plus 4 hours to freeze

These refreshing Strawberries and Cream Ice Pops are best made with a blender, but a food processor or handheld mixer will work, too. They taste so delicious, you won't believe they are quick and easy to prepare. You'll need 12 ice pop molds or 12 small paper cups and ice pop sticks.
Makes 12 pops

2 cups heavy (whipping) cream

8 ounces cream cheese, at room temperature

¼ cup sour cream

1 tablespoon freshly squeezed lemon juice

1½ cups sliced strawberries, divided

1 cup blueberries, divided

½ to ¾ cup granulated 1:1 sweetener

1. In a blender, blend the heavy cream, cream cheese, sour cream, and lemon juice until smooth. Add 1 cup strawberries, ½ cup blueberries, and the sweetener (more or less, depending on how sweet you like it) and blend until fully combined and smooth.

2. Spoon the remaining ½ cup strawberries and ½ cup blueberries into each ice pop mold, then pour in the cream mixture. Add the ice pop sticks. Freeze for 3 to 4 hours, or until frozen solid. Serve immediately after unmolding.

Per Serving (1 ice pop) Calories: 224; Total Fat: 22g; Total Carbs: 14g; Fiber: 1g; Net Carbs: 5g; Protein: 3g; Macros: Fat 88%/Protein 5%/Carbs 7%

Coconut-Lime Panna Cotta

Prep time: 10 minutes, plus 30 minutes to cool and 4 hours to chill
Cook time: 5 minutes

This panna cotta is bursting with tart lime and sweet coconut. Treat your-self to this simple and refreshing dessert any time you need something a little tropical. Top your panna cotta with a few fresh blueberries and some whipped cream for an extra-fancy treat. **Serves 4**

Coconut oil, for greasing

2 tablespoons unflavored powdered gelatin

3 tablespoons cold water

1 (13.5-ounce) can full-fat coconut milk

3 to 5 tablespoons granulated 1:1 sweetener

1 teaspoon grated lime zest

1 tablespoon freshly squeezed lime juice

½ teaspoon vanilla extract

⅛ teaspoon kosher salt

1. Grease four ramekins with coconut oil and set aside.

2. In a small bowl, soften the gelatin in the cold water and set aside.

3. In a medium saucepan, heat the coconut milk over medium heat until it's boiling. Reduce the heat and simmer for a couple of minutes, or until the cream begins to thicken. While stirring, add the sweetener (more or less, depending on how sweet you like it), lime zest, lime juice, vanilla, and salt. Continue to stir to combine all the ingredi-ents. Remove from the heat and add the gelatin and water. Stir until the gelatin is dissolved.

4. Pour the mixture into the prepared ramekins and let cool at room temperature for about 30 minutes. Cover with plastic wrap and put in the refrigerator for at least 4 hours before unmolding.

5. To remove the panna cotta from the ramekins, dip the ramekins in a bowl of hot water to help loosen. Serve cold.

Per Serving Calories: 180; Total Fat: 17g; Total Carbs: 15g; Fiber: 1g; Net Carbs: 4g; Protein: 4g; Macros: Fat 85%/ Protein 9%/Carbs 6%

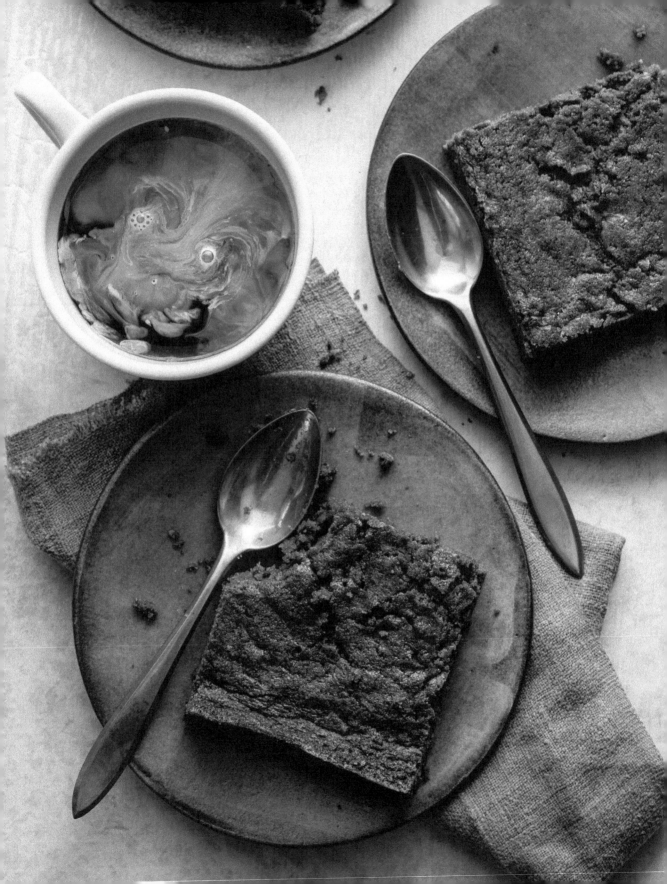

Classic Fudgy Brownies

Prep time: 10 minutes, plus 15 minutes to cool and 35 minutes to chill
Cook time: 30 minutes

These moist keto-friendly brownies will make you forget all about the kind made with flour and sugar. They'll keep in the freezer for up to 3 weeks.
Makes 16 brownies

4 ounces unsweetened baking chocolate, coarsely chopped

12 tablespoons (1½ sticks) unsalted butter, at room temperature

1 to 1¼ cups granulated 1:1 sweetener

3 eggs, at room temperature

1 teaspoon vanilla extract

1 cup almond flour, measured and sifted

1 teaspoon baking powder

¼ teaspoon kosher salt

1. Preheat the oven to 350°F. Line the bottom of an 8-inch square baking pan with parchment paper.

2. In a small microwave-safe bowl, melt the chocolate and butter together in the microwave in 30-second intervals until fully melted. Stir well and cool for 5 minutes.

3. In a medium bowl, whisk together the sweetener and the melted chocolate mixture. Using a hand-held mixer on medium-high, mix the eggs into the chocolate, one at a time, until well combined. Mix in the vanilla until the batter is smooth.

4. Whisk in the almond flour, baking powder, and salt, taking care not to overmix. Spread the batter in the prepared baking pan.

5. Bake for 20 to 25 minutes, until the center is just set but still jiggles.

6. Let cool on the rack for about 15 minutes. Refrigerate the cooled brownies for 30 to 35 minutes before cutting.

Per Serving (1 brownie) Calories: 175; Total Fat: 17g; Total Carbs: 16g; Fiber: 2g; Net Carbs: 2g; Protein: 4g; Macros: Fat 87%/Protein 9%/Carbs 4%

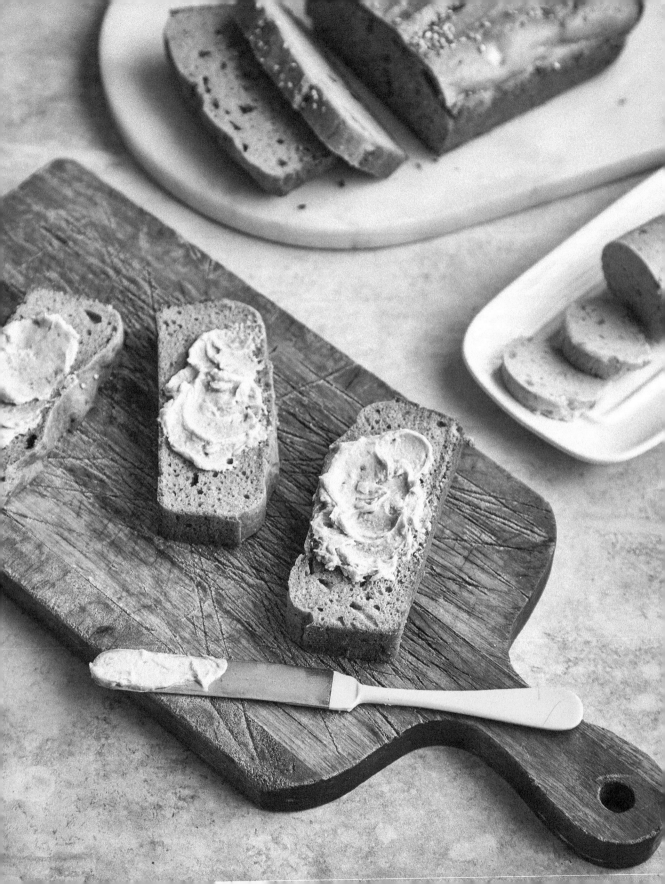

Keto Staples

Avocado Butter and Basic Sandwich Bread, pages180 and 188

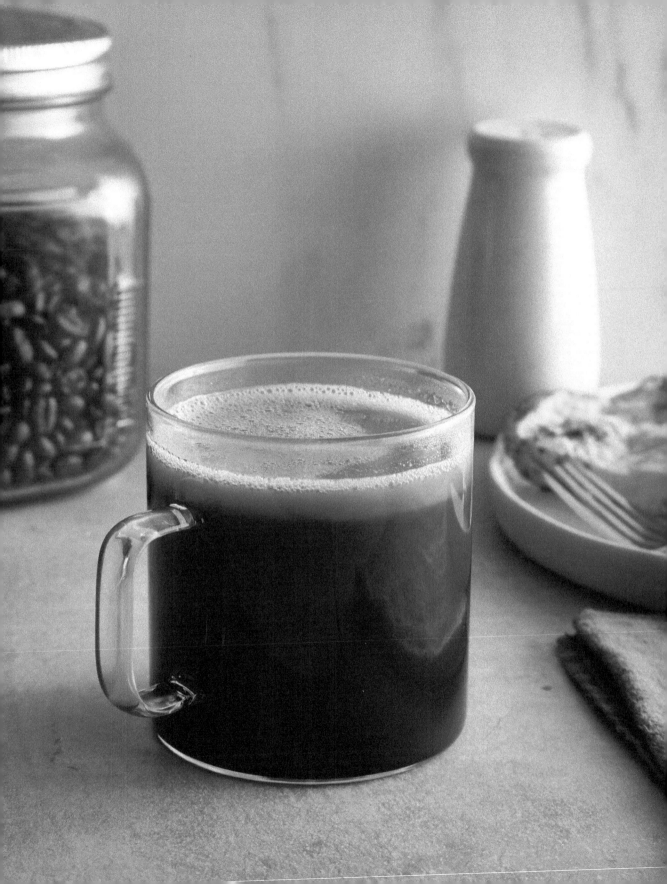

Fat Coffee

Prep time: 2 minutes Cook time: 5 minutes

This Fat Coffee may well become your morning keto staple. It will wake you up, keep your taste buds excited, and get you on your way to nutritional ketosis. Drinking one of these at least five mornings a week is a quick way to get a good amount of fat into your diet without spending the morning cooking. **Serves 1**

8 to 12 ounces black coffee

1 tablespoon butter

1 to 2 tablespoons MCT oil or powder or coconut oil

Pinch kosher salt

1. In a small saucepan, heat the coffee over medium heat. Stir in the butter, MCT oil, and salt.

2. Warm the mixture slowly, continuing to stir for 3 to 4 minutes. Serve warm.

Tip: If your coffee is still hot from the coffee maker, you can stir in the butter and oil right in your mug.

Per Serving Calories: 210; Total Fat: 26g; Total Carbs: 2g; Fiber: 1g; Net Carbs: 1g; Protein: <1g; Macros: Fat 99%/ Protein 0%/Carbs 1%

Three-Minute Mayo

Prep time: 3 minutes

There is nothing like making your own mayo. The ingredients are clean and fresh, and the flavor is delicious. Be sure to use mild avocado oil for this mayo and not olive oil. It will keep in the refrigerator for up to 4 days. To spice things up a bit, stir a few teaspoons of sriracha or adobo sauce from a can of chipotle peppers into the finished mayo. **Makes about 1 cup**

1 egg

1 egg yolk

2 teaspoons freshly squeezed lemon juice

1½ teaspoons Dijon mustard

1 or 2 garlic cloves, chopped

½ to ¾ teaspoon kosher salt

1 cup avocado oil

1. In a blender, combine the egg, yolk, lemon juice, mustard, garlic, and salt .

2. With the blender running on medium to medium-high, slowly stream in the avocado oil, blending until all the oil is fully incorporated and the mixture is thick, 1 to 2 minutes.

Tip: This fresh mayo uses raw eggs, so I like to use the freshest I have available. But if you're worried about consuming undercooked or raw eggs, use eggs that have been pasteurized in the shell.

Per Serving (1 tablespoon) Calories: 128; Total Fat: 14g; Total Carbs: <1g; Fiber: 0g; Net Carbs: <1g; Protein: 1g; Macros: Fat 99%/Protein 1%/Carbs 0%

Blender Hollandaise

Prep time: 3 minutes Cook time: 5 minutes

Rich and velvety, this easy hollandaise sauce is foolproof and comes together in just minutes in the blender. Use this lemony sauce as the finishing touch on broccoli, Brussels sprouts, asparagus, or over poached eggs for a Bacon-Avocado Benedict (page 33). **Makes about ¾ cup**

3 egg yolks, at room temperature

⅛ teaspoon kosher salt

Pinch cayenne pepper

1 tablespoon freshly squeezed lemon juice

8 tablespoons (1 stick) butter, cut into pieces

1. In a blender, combine the egg yolks, salt, cayenne pepper, and lemon juice.

2. In a small saucepan, melt the butter and heat until bubbly and foamy.

3. Blend the egg yolk mixture on high for a few seconds. Then, with the blender on high, remove the fill cap in the lid and slowly, in a thin stream, pour in the hot butter.

4. Taste the sauce and add more salt and lemon juice as needed. Serve immediately.

Tip: For a chipotle variation, add 2 to 3 teaspoons of adobo sauce from a can of chipotle peppers packed in adobo. Spoon the chipotle peppers into mounds onto a baking sheet and freeze, then put them in zip-top bags to use later.

Tip: For a dessert rendition, omit the salt and cayenne pepper. In step 1, add ½ teaspoon of vanilla extract, 3 tablespoons of powdered 1:1 sweetener, and ¼ cup of heavy cream to the egg yolks. Proceed with the instructions as written. Serve over berries.

Per Serving (1 tablespoon) Calories: 80; Total Fat: 9g; Total Carbs: <1g; Fiber: 0g; Net Carbs: <1g; Protein: 1g; Macros: Fat 99%/Protein 1%/Carbs 0%

Avocado Butter

Prep time: 5 minutes, plus 1 hour to chill

There's a ton of incredible flavor packed into this easy Avocado Butter. It's perfect for adding healthy fat to lean protein and dresses up anything from grilled steak and chicken to fish and shrimp. For the best results, use nicely ripe avocados. This will keep in the freezer for up to 1 week. **Makes 1 cup**

8 tablespoons (1 stick) butter, at room temperature

½ cup mashed avocado

2 tablespoons freshly squeezed lime juice

2 tablespoons finely chopped fresh cilantro

2 garlic cloves, finely minced

½ teaspoon ground cumin

½ teaspoon kosher salt

¼ teaspoon freshly ground black pepper

1. In a medium bowl, combine the butter and avocado and smash with a fork or potato masher until smooth. For a smoother butter, this step can also be done in a food processor. Stir in the lime juice, cilantro, garlic, cumin, salt, and pepper.

2. Spoon the mixture onto a piece of plastic wrap and shape it into a log. Refrigerate until firm, about 1 hour, then slice.

Tip: When shopping for avocados, remove the stem from the avocado. If it's barely green, the avocado is perfectly ripe. If it's missing or brown, the avocado is overripe.

Per Serving (1 tablespoon) Calories: 64; Total Fat: 7g; Total Carbs: 1g; Fiber: 1g; Net Carbs: 0g; Protein: <1g; Macros: Fat 100%/Protein 0%/Carbs 0%

Ranch Dressing

Prep time: 10 minutes

This homemade Ranch Dressing is a staple in our refrigerator and tastes better than anything you'll get out of a bottle. Drizzle it over a salad or use as a dip for veggies, wings, and more. It's best prepared in advance, if you have the time. It will keep in the refrigerator for up to 4 days. **Makes 1½ cups**

½ cup keto-friendly mayonnaise or Three-Minute Mayo (page 178)

¼ cup sour cream

1 garlic clove, grated or finely minced

¼ teaspoon onion powder

1 teaspoon dried parsley

1 teaspoon dried chives

¼ teaspoon Italian seasoning

½ teaspoon Worcestershire sauce

¼ teaspoon kosher salt

¼ teaspoon freshly ground black pepper

2 to 3 tablespoons unsweetened plain almond milk

1. In a medium bowl, whisk together the mayonnaise, sour cream, garlic, onion powder, parsley, chives, Italian seasoning, Worcestershire sauce, salt, and pepper.

2. To thin the dressing, add almond milk, 1 tablespoon at a time, until it reaches your desired consistency.

Tip: For an avocado variation, using a food processor or blender, process the ingredients with half of a medium avocado. The avocado will thicken the dressing significantly, so thin as desired with additional almond milk. Or for blue cheese, stir in ⅓ cup of crumbled blue cheese and thin as desired.

Per Serving (1 tablespoon) Calories: 39; Total Fat: 4g; Total Carbs: <1g; Fiber: 0g; Net Carbs: 0g; Protein: <1g; Macros: Fat 100%/Protein 0%/Carbs 0%

Creamy Feta Dressing

Prep time: 5 minutes

Creamy Feta Dressing literally takes minutes to whip up and tastes a million times better than the bottled or packaged stuff. It is great on anything from a simple dinner salad to a Cobb or Southwest salad. You can even use it in as a dip for veggies. It will keep in the refrigerator for up to 4 days.
Makes 1½ cups

½ cup sour cream

⅔ cup keto-friendly mayonnaise or Three-Minute Mayo (page 178)

⅓ cup unsweetened plain almond milk

½ teaspoon paprika

¼ teaspoon ground cumin

¼ teaspoon freshly ground black pepper

1 garlic clove, minced

⅓ cup crumbled feta cheese

In a bowl, whisk together the sour cream, mayonnaise, almond milk, paprika, cumin, pepper, garlic, and feta until smooth.

Per Serving (1 tablespoon) Calories: 60; Total Fat: 6g; Total Carbs: <1g; Fiber: 0g; Net Carbs: <1g; Protein: 1g; Macros: Fat 99%/Protein 1%/Carbs 0%

Quick Marinara Sauce

Prep time: 5 minutes Cook time: 30 minutes

Full of Italian flavor, this richly seasoned tomato sauce is great to have on hand for quick weeknight dinners, whether as a dip for your favorite meatballs or Herbed Mozzarella Sticks (page 45) or to use in recipes like Pepperoni Pizza Rolls (page 52) or One-Pan Chicken Parmesan (page 122). It will keep in the refrigerator for up to 4 days or in the freezer for up to 1 month. **Makes 3 cups**

2 tablespoons extra-virgin olive oil

1/3 cup diced onion

3 garlic cloves, finely minced

2 (14-ounce) cans crushed tomatoes

1/4 cup water

1 1/4 teaspoons dried basil

1 teaspoon dried parsley

1/2 teaspoon dried oregano

1 teaspoon granulated 1:1 sweetener

1 teaspoon kosher salt

1/4 teaspoon freshly ground black pepper

1. In a medium saucepan, heat the olive oil over medium heat and add the onion. Cook the onion for about 5 minutes, or until translucent. Add the garlic and cook for another minute.

2. Add the tomatoes, water, basil, parsley, oregano, sweetener, salt, and pepper and bring to a boil. Reduce the heat to low and simmer, uncovered, for about 20 minutes, stirring often.

3. Taste the sauce and adjust the salt and sweetener as desired.

Tip: I like to freeze marinara sauce in ice cube trays, and then store the frozen cubes in a zip-top bag for use when I need them. This enables you to thaw just as much as you need to for your recipe without wasting anything.

Per Serving Calories: 92; Total Fat: 5g; Total Carbs: 13g; Fiber: 3g; Net Carbs: 9g; Protein: 3g; Macros: Fat 49%/ Protein 13%/Carbs 38%

Easy Alfredo Sauce

Prep time: 5 minutes Cook time: 10 minutes

Rich, creamy, and so delicious, this simple Alfredo sauce is addictive, whether it's drizzled over broccoli, poured over chicken, used as the sauce for a white pizza, or tossed with zucchini noodles. This recipe makes quite a bit of sauce, and it's great to have on hand for quick meal prep. It will keep in the refrigerator for up to 5 days. **Makes 2 cups**

8 tablespoons (1 stick) butter

2 garlic cloves, finely minced

1½ cups heavy (whipping) cream

4 ounces cream cheese, at room temperature

1½ cups grated Parmesan cheese

¼ teaspoon freshly ground black pepper

1 tablespoon chopped fresh parsley (optional)

Kosher salt

1. In a medium saucepan, melt the butter over medium heat. Add the garlic and cook for 1 minute. Whisk in the heavy cream and cream cheese, continuing to whisk until the cream cheese is melted and the mixture comes to a simmer.

2. Remove from the heat and whisk in the Parmesan cheese until smooth. Stir in the pepper and parsley (if using). Taste and add salt, if desired.

Tip: Alfredo sauce tends to separate when reheated too quickly, so to reheat, heat it very slowly in a small saucepan over low heat, whisking constantly. Do not let it simmer or boil.

Per Serving (1 tablespoon) Calories: 96; Total Fat: 9g; Total Carbs: 1g; Fiber: 0g; Net Carbs: 1g; Protein: 2g; Macros: Fat 84%/Protein 8%/Carbs 8%

Cheesy Crackers

Prep time: 15 minutes Cook time: 35 minutes

Usually on a keto diet, people really miss bread and crackers. Made with cheese and almond flours, these simple crackers will satisfy those cravings. **Makes 55 to 60 crackers**

1¾ cups grated Parmesan cheese

1½ cups almond flour, plus more as needed

½ teaspoon kosher salt

½ teaspoon garlic powder

1 egg

2 tablespoons butter, melted

1. Preheat the oven to 300°F. Line a large baking sheet with parchment paper.

2. In a medium microwave-safe bowl, heat the Parmesan cheese in the microwave in 30-second increments until melted, stirring between each cycle.

3. Add the flour, salt, garlic powder, and egg to the cheese mixture. Stir quickly until a dough forms. If the batter seems too sticky, add more almond flour until it is no longer sticky.

4. Place the dough on a floured surface (or on a piece of parchment paper) and roll it out to ⅛ inch thick. Cut the dough into 1-inch squares and use a spatula to carefully transfer the crackers to the prepared baking sheet. Brush the butter across the top of each cracker.

5. Bake the crackers for 25 to 30 minutes, or until the tops are slightly browned. Remove from the oven and cool on the baking sheet.

Per Serving (5 crackers) Calories: 179; Total Fat: 15g; Total Carbs: 5g; Fiber: 2g; Net Carbs: 3g; Protein: 8g; Macros: Fat 75%/Protein 18%/Carbs 7%

Keto Dough

Prep time: 10 minutes Cook time: 2 minutes

This mozzarella-based dough is super versatile and can be used for both sweet and savory recipes with simple changes. From pizza, pigs in a blanket, and cheesy bread sticks to cinnamon rolls and keto crackers, this quick dough is all you need. You're limited only by your imagination.
Makes 12 servings

¾ cup almond flour

3 tablespoons coconut flour

2 teaspoons baking powder

¼ teaspoon kosher salt

2 cups grated mozzarella cheese

¼ cup cream cheese

2 eggs, lightly beaten

1. In a small bowl, combine the almond flour, coconut flour, baking powder, and salt.

2. In a large microwave-safe bowl, combine the mozzarella and cream cheeses. Microwave on high for 1 to 2 minutes, checking and stirring every 30 minutes, until melted and smooth.

3. Pour the almond flour mixture into the cheese mixture, add the eggs, and stir to combine. Use your hands as needed to work all the ingredients together until thoroughly incorporated.

4. Shape the dough into a ball and place it on a sheet of parchment paper. Cover with another piece of parchment and roll out according to the recipe instructions.

5. Store the prepared dough in the refrigerator for up to 4 days. Let it come to room temperature or warm for a few seconds in the microwave to use.

Italian Variation: Add ½ teaspoon of granulated garlic and ½ teaspoon of Italian seasoning to the almond flour mixture in step 1 and prepare as directed.

Sweet Variation: Add 2 tablespoons of powdered 1:1 sweetener to the almond flour mixture in step 1 and prepare as directed.

Pizza Crust: Roll the dough between two pieces of parchment paper to about ¼ inch thick, prick all over with a fork, and transfer to a baking sheet lined with parchment. Bake at 425°F for 10 to 12 minutes, or until golden, then add the desired toppings and bake until the cheese is melted and bubbly.

Keto Crackers: Divide the dough in half and roll one piece of dough between two pieces of parchment paper to about ⅛ inch thick. Brush with melted garlic butter, cut into squares with a pizza cutter, separate, and bake on a baking sheet lined with parchment at 325°F for 20 to 22 minutes, or until golden. Cool in the pan.

Per Serving Calories: 136; Total Fat: 11g; Total Carbs: 4g; Fiber: 1g; Net Carbs: 3g; Protein: 7g; Macros: Fat 73%/ Protein 20%/Carbs 7%

Basic Sandwich Bread

Prep time: 10 minutes, plus 40 minutes to cool Cook time: 40 minutes

This recipe makes a light, fluffy bread that is perfect for slicing, toasting, and of course, sandwiches. It freezes beautifully, so you can always have some on hand for when the cravings hit. Store any leftovers in the refrigerator for up to 7 days. **Makes 12 slices**

4 tablespoons (½ stick) unsalted butter, at room temperature, plus more for greasing

1¼ cups almond flour, sifted

1 tablespoon psyllium husk powder

2 teaspoons baking powder

½ teaspoon kosher salt

1 tablespoon granulated 1:1 sweetener

3½ ounces (about 7 tablespoons) cream cheese, at room temperature

4 eggs, at room temperature

2 tablespoons sesame seeds (optional)

1. Preheat the oven to 350°F. Grease a 9-by-5-inch loaf pan with butter.

2. In a medium bowl, combine the almond flour, psyllium husk powder, baking powder, and salt. Set aside.

3. Using a handheld mixer on medium-high speed in a large bowl, blend the butter and sweetener. Add the cream cheese and mix until well combined. Add the eggs, one at a time, making sure to mix well after each addition. Add the dry ingredients to the wet ingredients, and mix well until the batter is fully combined.

4. Spread the batter in the prepared loaf pan, then sprinkle the sesame seeds on top (if using). Bake the bread for 30 to 40 minutes, or until golden brown. The bread will be done when a toothpick inserted into the center comes out clean.

5. Let cool for about 10 minutes before removing from the pan. Place on a wire rack to cool for another 20 to 30 minutes before slicing.

Per Serving (1 slice) 156; Total Fat: 14g; Total Carbs: 5g; Fiber: 2g; Net Carbs: 2g; Protein: 5g; Macros: Fat 81%/ Protein 13%/Carbs 6%

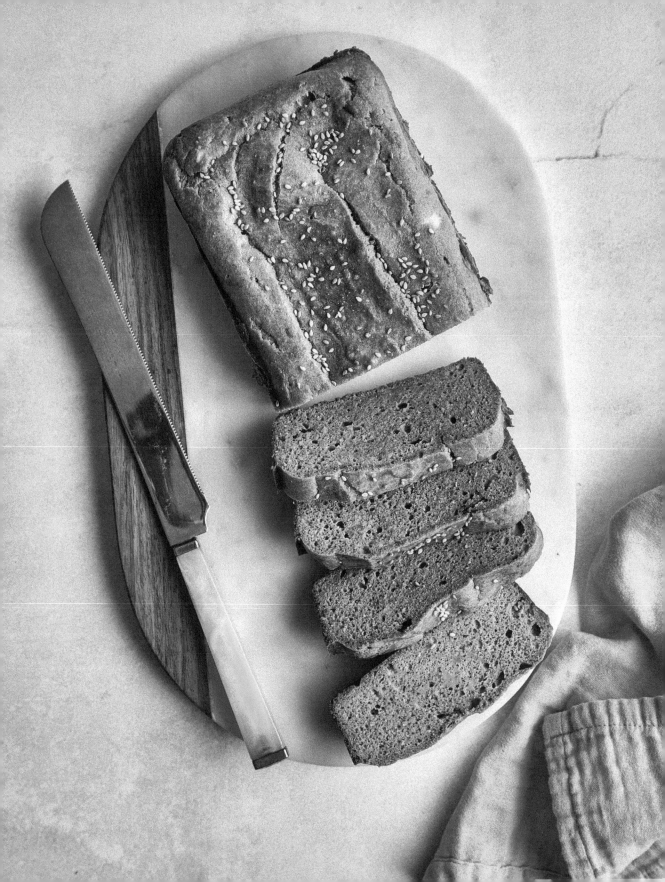

Strawberry Chia Jam

Prep time: 5 minutes Cook time: 10 minutes

This thick, fruity jam is the perfect spread for keto toast or biscuits, and makes the ideal topping for low-carb pancakes, waffles, ice cream, and anything else you might want to slather with strawberry jam. This will keep in the refrigerator for up to 1 week or in the freezer for up to 1 month.
Makes 1 cup

1 pound fresh or frozen strawberries, trimmed and quartered

3 tablespoons water

1 tablespoon freshly squeezed lemon juice

⅓ cup granulated 1:1 sweetener

1½ tablespoons chia seeds

1. In a medium saucepan, combine the strawberries, water, and lemon juice over medium heat and cook for 7 to 10 minutes, breaking the berries apart as they cook.

2. Add the sweetener and continue to cook for another 1 to 2 minutes, or until the sweetener is dissolved. Carefully taste the strawberry mixture and add more sweetener, if desired. Stir in the chia seeds and remove from the heat.

3. When cool, pour the mixture into a glass jar or other container, cover, and refrigerate.

Tip: The strawberries in this recipe can be swapped for any low-carb berries. Raspberries, blackberries, blueberries, and even dewberries will be fantastic, but you may have to adjust the amount of sweetener according to the sweetness of the fruit and your personal taste.

Per Serving (1 tablespoon) Calories: 15; Total Fat: <1g; Total Carbs: 7g; Fiber: 1g; Net Carbs: 2g; Protein: <1g; Macros: Fat 0%/Protein 0%/Carbs 100%

Beef Bone Broth

Prep time: 10 minutes, plus 3 hours to chill Cook time: 8 to 24 hours

Bone broth is a staple of many people on the keto diet, who sip this intense, deeply flavored broth in a mug to get essential collagen, vitamins, minerals, and electrolytes. In addition to a very lengthy cook time at low heat, this recipe calls for apple cider vinegar, which breaks down the collagen within the bones and helps extract it. When searching for bones, the price will depend on what's in stock and freshest. I often shop in the frozen meat section, where beef bones are sold specifically for making soup and are a great savings over fresh bones. Ask the butcher where the frozen beef bones are located. **Serves 6 to 8**

3 to 4 pounds beef bones (oxtails, neck bones, short ribs, etc.)

1 tablespoon extra-virgin olive oil

2 medium carrots, peeled and roughly chopped

2 celery stalks, roughly chopped

1 medium white onion, unpeeled, quartered

4 garlic cloves, peeled and smashed

3 bay leaves

2 tablespoons apple cider vinegar

1 tablespoon kosher salt

10 cups water

1. Preheat the oven to 400°F. Line a large baking sheet with aluminum foil. Place the bones on the baking sheet and drizzle with the olive oil. Roast for 1 hour, turning the bones over halfway through.

2. Continue cooking the bones on the stovetop or in a slow cooker or multicooker according to the instructions that follow these steps.

3. When the soup is cooked, remove the bones from the pot or cooker with tongs. Strain the broth into a large bowl to remove the vegetables. Discard the bones and vegetables. Cool the broth to room temperature, then refrigerate for at least 3 hours.

4. When the soup gels, spoon or scrape off any fat that has risen to the top, and discard. Portion the broth into zip-top freezer bags or freezer-safe containers and store in the freezer for up to 5 months.

continued >

Stovetop: In a large stockpot with a lid, combine the roasted bones and the carrots, celery, onion, garlic, bay leaves, vinegar, and salt. Pour in the water; the bones and vegetables should be completely covered. Bring to a boil over high heat. Reduce the heat to low, cover, and simmer for 8 to 12 hours.

Slow Cooker: In a slow cooker, combine the roasted bones and the carrots, celery, onion, garlic, bay leaves, vinegar, and salt. Pour in the water; the bones and vegetables should be completely covered. Cover and turn to the high setting. When the water starts to boil, turn to the low setting and cook for 18 to 24 hours.

Multicooker: In a multicooker, combine the roasted beef bones and the carrots, celery, onion, garlic, bay leaves, vinegar, and salt. Pour in the water; the bones and vegetables should be completely covered. Seal the lid and turn the manual setting to high. Set the timer for 2 hours. Allow the pressure to release naturally.

Per Serving Calories: 58; Total Fat: 4g; Total Carbs: 2g; Fiber: 1g; Net Carbs: 1g; Protein: 3g; Macros: Fat 62%/Protein 21%/Carbs 17%

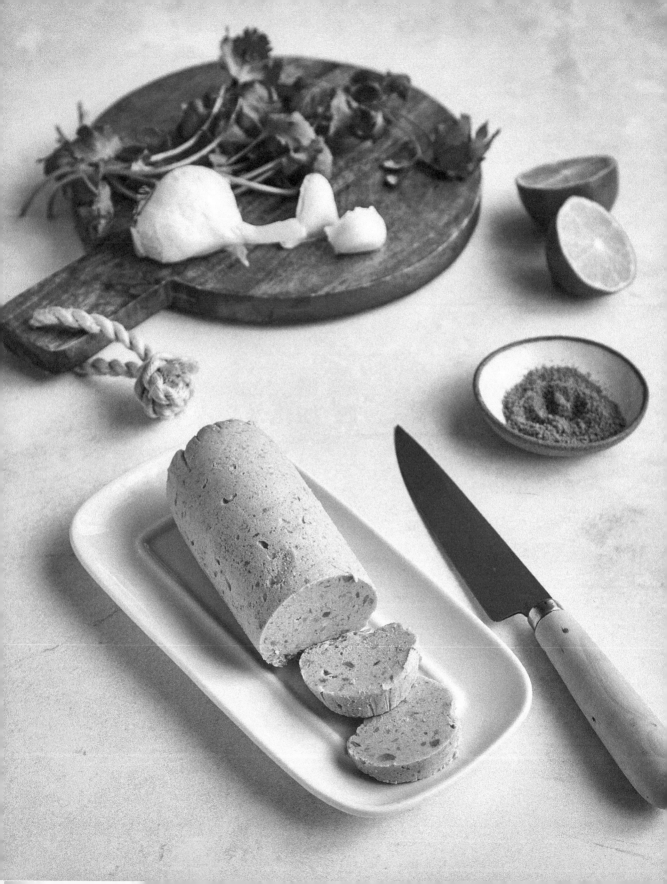

Measurement Conversions

Volume Equivalents

	U.S. Standard	U.S. Standard (ounces)	Metric (approximate)
Liquid	2 tablespoons	1 fl. oz.	30 mL
	¼ cup	2 fl. oz.	60 mL
	½ cup	4 fl. oz.	120 mL
	1 cup	8 fl. oz.	240 mL
	1½ cups	12 fl. oz.	355 mL
	2 cups or 1 pint	16 fl. oz.	475 mL
	4 cups or 1 quart	32 fl. oz.	1 L
	1 gallon	128 fl. oz.	4 L
Dry	⅛ teaspoon		0.5 mL
	¼ teaspoon		1 mL
	½ teaspoon		2 mL
	¾ teaspoon		4 mL
	1 teaspoon		5 mL
	1 tablespoon		15 mL
	¼ cup		59 mL
	⅓ cup		79 mL
	½ cup		118 mL
	⅔ cup		156 mL
	¾ cup		177 mL
	1 cup		235 mL
	2 cups or 1 pint		475 mL
	3 cups		700 mL
	4 cups or 1 quart		1 L
	½ gallon		2 L
	1 gallon		4 L

Oven Temperatures

Fahrenheit	Celsius (approximate)
250°F	120°C
300°F	150°C
325°F	165°C
350°F	180°C
375°F	190°C
400°F	200°C
425°F	220°C
450°F	230°C

Weight Equivalents

U.S. Standard	Metric (approximate)
½ ounce	15 g
1 ounce	30 g
2 ounces	60 g
4 ounces	115 g
8 ounces	225 g
12 ounces	340 g
16 ounces or 1 pound	455 g

Avocado Butter, page 180

Index

Acknowledgments

To Chase: None of this would be possible without you. You are my biggest cheerleader in life and in this whirlwind of a process. You're always more than willing to make the 65-mile trek to the store when I forget an ingredient, you never complain about my endless messes, and I can always count on your honest feedback. Thanks for always believing in me, even in the moments I doubt myself.

To my girls: My official taste testers, I love that you're both so willing to try new things and are always enthusiastic about testing my new creations. I couldn't do it without you!

To my extended ranch family: Thanks for always being willing testers, even when you don't know it! Your unending support means more than you know.

To my followers and friends: It's truly a gift to connect with all of you and hear your stories. I'm so honored that I get to be a small part of your journey, and I'll always be grateful for your support. All my best!

About the Author

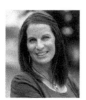

Emilie Bailey is a recipe developer, food photographer, author of *The Southern Keto Cookbook*, and the founder of *Tales of a Texas Granola Girl*, a recipe site specializing in gluten-free, low-carb, and keto comfort food dishes inspired by the Texas and Southern foods she grew up enjoying. After struggling with her weight and health for more than 20 years, she discovered the keto lifestyle and was able to drastically improve her symptoms and her overall health. She is passionate about helping others in their journey to better health by showing them just how delicious this lifestyle can be.

Emilie lives with her husband, The Cowboy, and their two girls on a busy game ranch in a tiny rural Texas community, and she also works as the ranch chef. You can browse through more of her keto recipes at TexasGranolaGirl.com.